EMT-INTERMEDIATE

PRETEST® SELF-ASSESSMENT AND REVIEW

EMT-INTERMEDIATE

PRETEST® SELF-ASSESSMENT AND REVIEW

Richard E.J. Westfal, M.D., F.A.C.E.P.
Associate Director
Department of Emergency Medicine
Saint Vincent's Hospital
New York, New York
Associate Professor
Department of Emergency Medicine
New York Medical College
Valhalla, New York

McGraw-Hill
Health Professions Division
PreTest® Series

New York   St. Louis   San Francisco   Auckland   Bogotá   Caracas   Lisbon   London   Madrid
Mexico City   Milan   Montreal   New Delhi   San Juan   Singapore   Sydney   Tokyo   Toronto

McGraw-Hill

*A Division of The **McGraw·Hill** Companies*

1 2 3 4 5 6 7 8 9 0   DOCDOC   9 9 8

ISBN 0-07-069636-5

This book was set in Times Roman by V&M Graphics.
The editors were John Dolan and Peter McCurdy.
The production supervisor was Helene G. Landers.
R.R. Donnelley & Sons was printer and binder.
The cover was designed by Li Chen Chang/Pinpoint.
The text was designed by Robert Freese.

This book is printed on acid-free paper.

CONTENTS

CONTENTS

PREFACE

Emergency Medical Technician–Intermediate: PreTest® Self-Assessment and Review has been developed to prepare entry level and refresher emergency medical technician–intermediate (EMT-I) students for National Registry, regional, state, and city examinations. This book also provides information to assist EMT-I instructors, course coordinators, and medical directors to assess the progress of their students.

The United States Department of Transportation instituted a new curriculum for a new level of emergency medical technician–intermediates in 1994. This intermediate level was designed to provide a connection between the emergency medical technician–basic (EMT-B) course and the emergency medical technician–paramedic (EMT-P) course. All emergency medical technician–intermediates will be required to pass a written qualifying examination in order to be certified or licensed to practice. The National Registry of Emergency Medical Technicians administers the EMT-I examinations, which are recognized by some of the states. Many states also administer their own entry examinations and require recertification examinations every two to five years.

The new curriculum is divided into major modules which include patient assessment, airway management and ventilation, medical emergencies, trauma, and other special considerations. This review text is divided into sections which correspond to each of the modules. Each section is further divided by the individual subjects contained in each module. The total number of review questions is about 400. The questions are distributed among all of the study topics but are particularly weighted towards more questions for the critical emergencies than to the minor illnesses and administrative areas. The division of the questions allows the student to evaluate his/her progress and to identify any areas of weakness. Students then may further review these areas and request additional help from their instructors.

Most of the questions are presented in the A-type multiple choice format. This format is the most frequently used format in state and national certifying exams. There is one correct answer and three distractors for each question. A brief explanation of the rationale for the correct answer is given for each question. The questions are referenced to information provided in the following textbooks: American Academy of Orthopaedic Surgeons' (A.A.O.S.) Emergency Care and Transportation of the Sick and Injured, Brady's Intermediate Emergency Care, Mosby's EMT–Intermediate Textbook, and McGraw-Hill's EMT–Basic: PreTest® Self-Assessment and Review. Each answer has a chapter reference for the corresponding material in the textbooks. This should assist students in studying areas where they may need improvement.

I hope that this text will assist each student in his/her pursuit of advancement in an emergency medical service career.

I would like to thank Peter McCurdy for his supervision of the editing of the text and my editor, John Dolan, for his consistent support and guidance.

Note

The bibliographic citations following each answer cite the publisher of the book first (Brady, AAOS, or Mosby) and the section or chapter (e.g., Patient Assessment or The Detailed Physical Exam) in that book in which relevant information can be found. For full book information on each citation, please see the Bibliography, on page 223.

EMT-INTERMEDIATE

PRETEST® SELF-ASSESSMENT AND REVIEW

ROLES AND RESPONSIBILITIES

In this chapter, you will review:

- EMT-I characteristics

- meaning of the EMT-I certification

- professional and ethical conduct of an EMT-I

ROLES AND RESPONSIBILITIES

Directions: Each item below contains four suggested responses. Select the **one best** response to each item.

1. All of the following are characteristics of the position of an EMT-Basic (EMT-B) EXCEPT

   (A) it includes 300–1600 hours of training
   (B) the training is based on the 1994 DOT Emergency Medical Technician-Basic Curriculum
   (C) training as an EMT-B is usually a prerequisite for advanced emergency medical service (EMS)-level training courses
   (D) basic skills and, in some communities, certain advanced skills must be learned

2. All of the following are characteristics which identify an EMT-Intermediate (EMT-I) EXCEPT

   (A) the position was created to span the gap between the EMT-B and the EMT-Paramedic (EMT-P)
   (B) examples of the EMT-I level include EMT-Cardiac, EMT-II, EMT-Advanced, EMT-Special Skills, and Cardiac Rescue Technician (CRT)
   (C) many states require an EMT-I to work under medical direction
   (D) an EMT-I is not responsible for overseeing expiration dates on medications or evaluating equipment for the proper function

3. All of the following are aspects of the EMT-P level of training EXCEPT

   (A) training usually goes 300–1600 hours beyond the EMT-B level

   (B) many colleges have a 2- or 4-year program in EMS, which includes EMT-P certification

   (C) an EMT-P never treats patients under standing orders, only under direct medical control by radio or telephone contact with a physician

   (D) EMT-P is the highest level of prehospital EMS provider

4. The role of an EMT-I is to provide

   (A) only prehospital basic life support

   (B) only prehospital advanced life support

   (C) basic and advanced life support only for medical emergencies

   (D) basic and advanced life support for medical and traumatic emergencies

5. All of the following are responsibilities of an EMT-I EXCEPT

   (A) ensuring his or her safety and that of his or her fellow workers

   (B) interacting with the First Responders already on the scene

   (C) throughout the call, maintaining control of the safety of the scene even after the police arrive

   (D) rapidly assessing and treating lifethreatening emergencies

6. Which of the following is the correct definition of certification, as in EMT-I certification?

   (A) The process of guaranteeing the record of an EMT-I's run report

   (B) The action of an agency or association to grant recognition to an individual who has met its qualifications

   (C) A government agency granting lifetime permission to practice in a medical field

   (D) The action by a federal agency to validate the expiration dates of drugs used by an EMT-I in the field

7. Which of the following is the correct definition of the term *licensure*?

   (A) A governmental agency grants permission for an individual to engage in an occupation after finding that he or she has attained the minimal degree of competency

   (B) An agency recognizes a person for passing a challenging examination

   (C) An agency recognizes the process of training by another state agency

   (D) A governmental agency has granted leeway for an individual to practice in a somewhat different manner than do others in the same field

8. Which of the following statements best describes the role of the National Registry of Emergency Medical Technicians (NREMT)?

(A) Provides a national referral list of certified EMT-Is for job placement

(B) Provides the only means for nationally certified EMT-Is to transfer their credentials from state to state

(C) Prepares and administers standardized examinations on a national basis and establishes the qualifications for registration as EMT-B, EMT-I, and EMT-P

(D) Provides licensing examinations for already certified EMT-Is

9. Which of the following is the correct meaning of EMT-I certification?

(A) Gives one the right to function as an EMT-I

(B) Guarantees reciprocity between states in regard to employment

(C) Documents that an EMT-I has demonstrated the minimum written and practical proficiency

(D) Guarantees one's eligibility to be selected immediately for employment

10. Which of the following is the best reason to keep one's EMT-I certification or licensure current?

(A) Employers often pay bonuses for keeping it current

(B) In most states it is legally required to maintain current certification in order to practice as an EMT-I

(C) It automatically makes one a candidate for an EMT-P training course

(D) It makes one an EMT-B practical skills instructor

11. All of the following are reasons why continuing medical education (CME) is important to the EMT-I EXCEPT

(A) most employers provide bonuses for doing so

(B) it helps assure high-quality patient care

(C) it helps prevent knowledge and skill erosion

(D) it helps keep an EMT-I up to date on new treatments and procedures

12. All of the following are benefits of subscribing to EMS professional journals EXCEPT

(A) it gives an EMT-I an opportunity to write articles about his or her experiences

(B) it is an excellent source of financial and tax advice

(C) it provides employment opportunities and a chance for professional advancement

(D) it provides job-related tips and announcements of upcoming conferences

13. All of the following are benefits of EMT-I teaching in the community EXCEPT

(A) acquiring CME credits

(B) keeping one's skills current

(C) establishing an EMT-I as a leader and resource in the community

(D) automatically allowing one to be selected for an EMT-P training course

14. Which of the following is the best definition of *ethics*?

    (A) The study of philosophy
    (B) The discipline dealing with differences between various cultures
    (C) The discipline dealing with what is good and bad
    (D) The discipline dealing with medical-legal issues

15. All of the following are parts of the definition of *professionalism* EXCEPT

    (A) a person who must be paid for his or her services
    (B) a person with certain skills and knowledge in a specific area
    (C) a person who conforms to standards of conduct in a specific area
    (D) a person who conforms to standards of performance in a specific area

16. All of the following are behaviors on the part of an EMT-I which are considered professional EXCEPT

    (A) quietly demanding respect from patients
    (B) demonstrating true concern for each patient
    (C) treating all patients with respect by addressing them by the proper name (e.g., Mr. Jones)
    (D) striving for personal improvement as an EMT-I by pursuing continuing education and reading EMS journals

17. All of the following are aspects of the appropriate professional appearance of an EMT-I EXCEPT

    (A) being well groomed
    (B) wearing appropriate jewelry, earrings, and necklaces
    (C) wearing an appropriate uniform
    (D) wearing personal protection apparel

18. All of the following are considered attributes of ethical conduct by an EMT-I EXCEPT

    (A) respecting patient confidentiality
    (B) providing services based on human need, unrestricted by race, nationality, creed, color, or status
    (C) maintaining professional knowledge and skills
    (D) delegating tasks to others regardless of their professional training or capabilities

19. All of the following are major purposes of the National Association of EMTs EXCEPT

    (A) serving the needs of EMTs
    (B) trying to restrict the hiring of EMTs by agencies other than the national organization
    (C) promoting the professional status of EMTs
    (D) encouraging the continuous upgrading of education and skills for EMTs

ROLES AND RESPONSIBILITIES

ANSWERS

1. **The answer is A.** (Mosby, *Roles and Responsibilities of EMT-I.*) (B), (C), and (D) are correct. (A) is incorrect because the EMT-B training course usually entails at least 110 hours of training, not 300–1600 hours.

2. **The answer is D.** (Brady, *Roles and Responsibilities of EMT-I.* Mosby, *Roles and Responsibilities of EMT-I.*) (A), (B), and (C) are correct. (D) is incorrect because an EMT-I is responsible for checking the expiration dates on medications and evaluating the proper function of equipment.

3. **The answer is C.** (Mosby, *Roles and Responsibilities of EMT-I.*) (A), (B), and (D) are correct. (C) is incorrect because an EMT-P usually provides advanced prehospital care through a combination of standing orders and direct medical control, depending on the EMS system.

4. **The answer is D.** (Mosby, *Roles and Responsibilities of EMT-I.*) (D) provides the correct definition of the role of an EMT-I. (A), (B), and (C) are all incorrect.

5. **The answer is C.** (Mosby, *Roles and Responsibilities of EMT-I.*) (A), (B), (D), establishing rapport and treating all patients with dignity and respect, driving an emergency vehicle safely, using protective equipment, communicating with the dispatchers and medical directors, gaining access to and trying to extricate entrapped patients, performing careful patient assessment and treating patients according to protocols, transporting patients to the correct destination, transferring patients safely and gently to the ambulance and the emergency department, running report documentation, preparing for the next call, assessing the effects of treatment, and recognizing when transport may not be necessary are some of the responsibilities of an EMT-I. (C) is incorrect because initially an EMT-I establishes scene safety. However, after the police arrive, they usually are responsible for scene safety.

6. The answer is B. (Mosby, *Roles and Responsibilities of EMT-I.*) (B) is correct. (A), (C), and (D) are incorrect.

7. The answer is A. (Mosby, *Roles and Responsibilities of EMT-I.*) (A) is the correct definition of licensure. (B), (C), and (D) provide incorrect definitions.

8. The answer is C. (Brady, *Roles and Responsibilities of EMT-I.*) (C) is correct. (A), (B), and (D) are all incorrect.

9. The answer is C. (Mosby, *Roles and Responsibilities of EMT-I.*) (C) is correct. (A) is incorrect because EMS employers may impose requirements for employment in addition to certification. (B) is incorrect because reciprocity between states varies from state to state. Many but not all states accept NREMT certification. (D) is incorrect because there are no guarantees of employment.

10. The answer is B. (Mosby, *Roles and Responsibilities of EMT-I.*) (B) is correct. (A), (C), and (D) are incorrect.

11. The answer is A. (Mosby, *Roles and Responsibilities of EMT-I.*) (B), (C), and (D) are correct. (A) is incorrect because employers do not give bonuses for participating in continuing medical education (CME).

12. The answer is B. (Mosby, *Roles and Responsibilities of EMT-I.* Brady, *Roles and Responsibilities of EMT-I.*) Professional journals provide excellent CME-related articles and information and describe the latest changes in the EMS industry. (B) is incorrect because giving financial and tax advice is not one of the functions of EMS journals.

13. The answer is D. (Mosby, *Roles and Responsibilities of EMT-I.*) (A), (B), and (C) are correct. (D) is incorrect because being active in EMT-I teaching may help better prepare an EMT-I as a student in an EMT-P training course but does not facilitate selection for such a course.

14. The answer is C. (Mosby, *Roles and Responsibilities of EMT-I.*) (C) is correct. (A), (B), and (D) are incorrect.

15. The answer is A. (Mosby, *Roles and Responsibilities of EMT-I.*) (B), (C), and (D) are all correct. (A) is incorrect because an EMT-I does not have to be paid in order to be professional.

16. The answer is A. (Mosby, *Roles and Responsibilities of EMT-I.*) (B), (C), and (D), appearance, general conduct, and demonstration of professional manner are all EMT-I behaviors that are considered professional. (A) is incorrect because an EMT-I gives respect to but does not demand respect from his or her patients.

17. The answer is B. (Mosby, *Roles and Responsibilities of EMT-I.*) (A), (C), and (D) are correct. (B) is incorrect because jewelry, earrings, and necklaces are not considered parts of the appropriate apparel for an EMT-I.

18. The answer is D. (Mosby, *Roles and Responsibilities of EMT-I.*) (D) is incorrect because the EMT-I often delegates tasks to others, based upon their professional training or capabilities. (A), (B), (C), upholding the law and doing one's duty as a citizen, assuming responsibility in defining and maintaining professional actions, maintaining awareness of EMT-related legislative matters, and working with other members of the EMS team are some of the attributes of ethical conduct by an EMT-I.

19. The answer is B. (Mosby, *Roles and Responsibilities of EMT-I.*) (A), (C), and (D) are correct. (B) is incorrect because the National Association of EMTs is not involved in the hiring of EMTs.

EMS SYSTEMS

In this chapter, you will review:

- access to the EMS system

- role of the EMT-I in the prehospital system

- the definition of medical direction

EMS SYSTEMS

Directions: Each item below contains four suggested responses. Select the **one best** response to each item.

20. Which of the following statements BEST explains why prehospital care is an extension of hospital care?

(A) Prehospital medications are the same as those used in the hospital

(B) Prehospital providers use medical phrases similar to those used in the hospital

(C) Although prehospital providers deliver the care, the legal responsibility falls on the medical direction physician, as is the case in the hospital

(D) Prehospital providers often use devices to draw blood that are the same as those used in the hospital

21. Which of the following emergently ill patients requires immediate transport to the hospital rather than an attempt at stabilization in the field?

(A) A 64-year-old patient with chest pain

(B) A 41-year-old patient with a stab wound to the chest

(C) A 23-year-old patient with asthma

(D) An 81-year-old patient with an infected foot

22. The provision of prehospital emergency medical care is part of the continuum of the emergency phase of hospital care. All of the following are examples of this continuum EXCEPT

(A) emergency medicine nurses

(B) emergency medicine physicians

(C) emergency medicine–based physician assistants, respiratory therapists, and radiology technicians

(D) emergency medicine dietitians

23. All of the following are ways of providing citizen access to the emergency medical system (EMS) EXCEPT

(A) dialing 911
(B) calling the police
(C) calling a volunteer ambulance service
(D) calling the mayor's office

24. All of the following are considered members of the EMS team EXCEPT

(A) First Responders
(B) EMT-Basics (EMT-Bs)
(C) EMT-Intermediates (EMT-Is)
(D) Emergency Department (ED) physician assistants

25. All of the following are components of an EMS system EXCEPT

(A) communications, administration, facilities, training
(B) medical direction, disaster linkage, research, transportation
(C) medical records, quality improvement, labor power, equipment and supplies
(D) pathology, morgue, laboratories, admitting office

26. In 1974 the General Services Administration established a set of standards for ambulance design. These standards are commonly referred to as

(A) KKK ambulance standards
(B) AAA ambulance standards
(C) EMS ambulance standards
(D) EMT ambulance standards

27. All EMS systems use a significant amount of supplies and equipment in a basic ambulance. Which of the following organizations has established the accepted minimal standard list of required supplies and equipment?

(A) American College of Surgeons
(B) American College of Emergency Physicians (ACEP)
(C) American College of University Professors
(D) National Association of EMS Physicians

28. All of the following are examples of EMS equipment which emergency departments usually store for the ambulance crew to return to pick up EXCEPT

(A) pneumatic antishock trousers
(B) long boards
(C) splints
(D) portable radios

29. Which of the following is the correct definition of *medical direction*?

(A) The telemetry orders given by physicians
(B) An EMS committee of physicians writing paramedic protocols
(C) A state committee of physicians writing new revisions of EMT curricula
(D) The medical supervision of an EMS system and the field performance of EMTs

30. Medical direction usually is defined as having two parts: on-line medical control and off-line medical control. The main component of on-line medical control is

(A) meeting the arriving EMS crew to review the care rendered
(B) the medical advice given by the EMS dispatchers
(C) after the EMT-I assesses the patient, he or she makes radio or telephone contact to receive medical instructions
(D) after the EMT-I completes the provision of emergent medical care, he or she transports the patient to an emergency department and reviews the care already rendered to the patient

31. Off-line medical direction involves all of the following EXCEPT

(A) administrative matters, including protocol development, training, and system design
(B) EMS physician participation in providing an actual review of prehospital care in the field and in the ED as well as participation in prehospital research studies
(C) retrospective review of actual prehospital care, quality control, and risk management
(D) radio communication with EMT-Is in the field

32. Which of the following is the BEST explanation for the importance of the medical community's role in overseeing prehospital care?

(A) An EMT-I's care in the field is an extension of hospital and physician services
(B) Federal laws mandate this relationship
(C) EMT-Is are not considered capable of providing independent care
(D) The medical community prefers to be in charge

33. In the delivery of prehospital care, a set of written policies and procedures for EMT-Is to follow is often referred to as

(A) rules and regulations
(B) bylaws
(C) protocols
(D) statutes

34. The actual provision of EMT-I treatments and procedures which can be completed before contacting medical direction is known as

(A) on-line medical control
(B) standing orders
(C) off-line medical control
(D) bylaws

35. Which of the following BEST describes the usual relationship between the physician on the radio and the EMT-I?

(A) The EMT-I evaluates the patient and then calls the physician on the radio for instructions before rendering certain care

(B) The EMT-I assesses the patient, provides complete basic and advanced prehospital care, and then calls the physician on the radio to review that care

(C) The EMT-I calls the physician on the radio en route to the patient to discuss possible treatment options before seeing the patient

(D) The physician on the radio initiates the call to the EMT-I after being told about the nature of the call from the EMS dispatcher

36. The individual physician who is responsible for medical direction in an EMS system is known as the

(A) physician in charge
(B) attending physician
(C) medical director
(D) dean

37. All of the following are parts of the process of quality improvement, which is the main responsibility of the medical director, EXCEPT

(A) attending statewide meetings on employment opportunities for medical directors
(B) reviewing ambulance run reports
(C) organizing continuing medical education
(D) taking corrective action when improper care has been rendered

38. All of the following are areas of concern when the medical director reviews ambulance run reports as part of quality improvement EXCEPT

(A) actual chart documentation
(B) response time data
(C) adherence of the EMT-I to protocols
(D) mileage on the ambulance

EMS SYSTEMS

A N S W E R S

20. The answer is C. (Mosby, *EMS Systems.*) (C) is correct. While (A), (B), and (D) describe situations that are often the same as in the hospital, they are not the best explanations why prehospital care is an extension of hospital care.

21. The answer is B. (Mosby, *EMS Systems.*) (B) is correct because trauma patients frequently require blood transfusions and hemorrhage control, which usually can be done only in an operating room at a hospital. (A), (C), and (D) all describe patients who should receive initial attempts at stabilization in the field.

22. The answer is D. (Mosby, *EMS Systems.*) (A), (B), and (C) are all correct because these professionals often continue the provision of emergency medical care that was initiated in the field by prehospital providers. (D) is incorrect because while a patient's dietary needs are often very important during his or her hospitalization and postdischarge care, they are not considered part of the continuum of prehospital emergency care.

23. The answer is D. (Mosby, *EMS Systems.*) Dialing the fire department, calling 911, calling the police, and calling private ambulance services are some of the mechanisms used in various communities to provide citizen access to the EMS service. Calling the mayor's office is not a commonly used mechanism to bring emergency medical care.

24. The answer is D. (Mosby, *EMS Systems.*) The first three groups of professionals, along with EMT-Paramedics (EMT-Ps), are considered members of the EMS team. (D) is incorrect because ED physician assistants are members of the emergency department team, not the EMS team.

25. The answer is D. (Mosby, *EMS Systems.*) (A), (B), (C), funding, consumer information and education, critical care units, public safety agencies, and mutual aid are all components of an EMS system. (D) is incorrect because these functions are all components of a hospital system but usually are not considered components of an EMS system.

26. **The answer is A.** (Brady, *Emergency Medical Services Systems.*) (A) is correct. In 1980, 1985, and 1990 there were updated revisions of the KKK standards. (B), (C), and (D) are incorrect.

27. **The answer is A.** (Mosby, *EMS Systems.*) (A) is the correct answer. (B), (C), and (D) are all incorrect. However, while (B) and (D) list organizations which are involved in EMS systems and the delivery of prehospital emergency medical care, the American College of University Professors. (C) has nothing to do with these functions.

28. **The answer is D.** (Mosby, *EMS Systems.*) (A), (B), and (C) are correct because these are pieces of equipment which are frequently attached to emergently ill patients and cannot be immediately detached. (D) is incorrect because portable radios are key pieces of communication equipment which an ambulance crew would never leave at the ED.

29. **The answer is D.** (Mosby, *EMS Systems.*) (D) is the correct definition. (A), (B), and (C) are incorrect because each identifies a component of medical direction, while (D) provides the full definition.

30. **The answer is C.** (Mosby, *EMS Systems.*) (C) is correct. (A), (B), and (D) are incorrect.

31. **The answer is D.** (Mosby, *EMS Systems.*) (A), (B), and (C) are aspects of off-line medical direction. (D) is incorrect because radio communication is part of on-line medical direction.

32. **The answer is A.** (Mosby, *EMS Systems.*) (A) is correct. (B), (C), and (D) are incorrect.

33. **The answer is C.** (Mosby, *EMS Systems.*) (C) is correct. (A), (B), and (D) are incorrect.

34. **The answer is B.** (Mosby, *EMS Systems.*) (B) is correct. (A), (C), and (D) are incorrect.

35. **The answer is A.** (Mosby, *EMS Systems.*) (A) is correct. (B), (C), and (D) are all incorrect.

36. **The answer is C.** (Mosby, *EMS Systems.*) (C) is correct even though this person may choose to delegate certain aspects of his or her role to others. (A), (B), and (D) are incorrect.

37. **The answer is A.** (Mosby, *EMS Systems.*) (B), (C), and (D) are parts of the quality improvement responsibilities of an EMS medical director. (A) is incorrect.

38. **The answer is D.** (Mosby, *EMS Systems.*) (A), (B), and (C) are correct. (D) is incorrect because the mileage on the ambulance is not a matter of concern to the medical director when he or she is performing a quality improvement review of the ambulance run report.

MEDICAL-LEGAL ISSUES

In this chapter, you will review:

- the Good Samaritan laws/state EMS statutes
- negligence
- types of consent

MEDICAL-LEGAL ISSUES

Directions: Each item below contains four suggested responses. Select the **one best** response to each item.

39. A *tort* is defined as

    (A) a law involving marital relations

    (B) the actual breaking of a law which damages the public

    (C) breach of a legal duty or obligation resulting in a physical, mental, or financial injury

    (D) the actual crime and punishment involved in committing an offense

40. Match the following categories with the correct descriptions:

    (A) Good samaritan act/civil immunity _____

    (B) DNR order _____

    (C) State motor vehicle codes _____

    (D) State medical practice act _____

    (E) State EMS statutes _____

      1. Physician's order not to resuscitate a patient

      2. Actual rules and regulations governing the practice of EMS providers

      3. Protects an individual acting at the scene of an emergency if he or she acts in good faith, is not negligent, acts within the scope of practice, and does not bill for services

      4. Statutes regarding the operation of emergency vehicles

      5. Defines an EMT-I's scope of practice, assessment, and treatment skills permitted to be performed

41. All of the following are parts of good samaritan laws EXCEPT

   (A) protecting people from liability for assisting at the scene of a medical emergency
   (B) protecting people who act in good faith even if they perform a negligent act
   (C) protecting people in an emergency as long as they perform acts within their scope of training
   (D) protecting prehospital personnel who are paid to provide emergent care

42. All of the following are situations an EMT-I must report to the appropriate legal authorities EXCEPT

   (A) suspected child abuse
   (B) suspected elder abuse
   (C) suspected rape
   (D) suspected noncompliance with medications

43. Which of the following is the best definition of *negligence,* as in medical liability?

   (A) Conduct that falls below the standard of care
   (B) Conduct which is personally upsetting to the patient and/or the patient's family
   (C) Failure to arrive at work on time
   (D) The act of leaving a lecture early

44. Medical liability is considered the same as which of the following?

   (A) Negligence
   (B) Inappropriate verbal communication
   (C) Inappropriate professional appearance
   (D) Perjury

45. All of the following are ways in which an EMT-I has a duty to act EXCEPT

   (A) a signed contract to provide EMS services
   (B) being dispatched to a call
   (C) arriving at the scene of a call
   (D) seeing a sick patient while off duty

46. The four elements required to prove negligence include all of the following EXCEPT

   (A) the act or omission must have been an element of the EMT-I's duty to act
   (B) the act or omission must have been above the standard of care
   (C) an injury must have occurred to the patient
   (D) the act or omission must have been the proximate (direct) cause of the injury

47. Match each of the following types of consent with the correct definition:

   (A) Consent _____
   (B) Expressed consent _____
   (C) Implied consent _____
   (D) Informed consent _____

   1. The benefits and risks of treatment must be stated so that the patient understands them
   2. The granting of permission to treat
   3. Assuming that the patient would want lifesaving treatment if he or she could consent to it
   4. The patient gives consent verbally, nonverbally, or in writing

48. To properly obtain informed consent, all of the following must be presented to an alert patient with a nonurgent problem EXCEPT

- (A) the EMT-I's assessment of the medical condition
- (B) the type of treatment being considered and why
- (C) the exact doses and references for the use of certain medications
- (D) an explanation of the benefits and risks of accepting or refusing examination, care, or transportation

49. Match the following terms with the correct definitions:

- (A) Abandonment _____
- (B) Assault _____
- (C) Battery _____
- (D) False imprisonment _____
- (E) Libel _____
- (F) Slander _____

1. Intentional and unjustifiable imprisonment of a person against his or her will
2. Injury of a person's character, name, or reputation through false or malicious writings
3. EMT-I touches and injures a patient without that person's consent
4. A patient fears that an EMT-I will cause him or her bodily harm without the patient's consent
5. Verbally making false statements which defame and damage another person's reputation
6. Negligence which occurs when an EMT-I terminates a relationship with a patient without providing continuity of care

50. The use of force and restraint to protect an EMT-I, a patient, and/or a third party frequently occurs in all of the following situations EXCEPT

- (A) a patient who is verbally abusive to the EMT-I
- (B) a patient with psychiatric problems
- (C) a patient who abuses alcohol and/or drugs
- (D) a patient who is suicidal

51. In considering the use of force and restraint to protect a patient, an EMT-I, and/or any third party, it is important to be familiar with which of the following?

- (A) Tort law on this topic
- (B) Federal and municipal good samaritan laws
- (C) A good malpractice attorney
- (D) The state laws on this subject

52. All of the following are important facts for an EMT-I who wants to comply with COBRA patient transfer requirements EXCEPT

   (A) an unstable patient is not to be transferred unless the patient or his or her representative so requests or if appropriate treatment facilities are unavailable at the initial institution

   (B) before transfer, all patients must be stabilized unless the risk of stabilizing outweighs the benefit of transferring a patient to a specialty center

   (C) knowledge that COBRA stands for the Cooperative Only Because of Retribution Act of 1985

   (D) the EMT-I and the hospital are potentially liable once the patient is in a hospital-owned ambulance, if that patient is not appropriately transported to the hospital

53. All of the following are examples of the importance of an EMT-I accurately and exactly documenting the medical record EXCEPT

   (A) child abuse
   (B) crime scene
   (C) inventory checklists
   (D) physician at the scene requesting to be in charge

MEDICAL-LEGAL ISSUES

ANSWERS

39. The answer is C. (Mosby, *Medical/Legal Considerations.*) (C) is correct. Tort law involves a plaintiff, or injured person, filing a lawsuit against a defendant, or person accused of committing a breach of duty. (A) is not the correct definition. (B) and (D) relate to criminal law, not tort law.

40. Answers. (Mosby, *Medical/Legal Considerations.* Brady*, Medical-Legal Considerations of Emergency Care.*)
(A) 3
(B) 1
(C) 4
(D) 5
(E) 2

41. The answer is B. (Brady, *Medical-Legal Considerations of Emergency Care.*) (A), (C), and (D) are correct statements. (B) is incorrect because one is not protected if one performs a negligent act.

42. The answer is D. (Mosby, *Medical/Legal Considerations.*) (A), (B), (C), gunshot wounds, and animal bites are some of the mandatory reportable incidents. EMT-Is must familiarize themselves with any other requirements in their state, city, or emergency medical services (EMS) systems. (C) is incorrect because it is not necessary to report noncompliance with medications to any legal authorities. However, this represents very important medical information which should be recorded on the chart and communicated to medical control and/or the receiving emergency department.

43. **The answer is A.** (Mosby, *Medical/Legal Considerations.*) (A) is the correct definition. (B), (C), and (D) may all constitute negligent acts, but they are not related to the definition of *negligence.*

44. **The answer is A.** (Mosby, *Medical/Legal Considerations.*) *Negligence* is synonymous with *medical liability.* The other terms are not.

45. **The answer is D.** (Mosby, *Medical/Legal Considerations.*) (A), (B), and (C) are correct. (D) is incorrect because when one is off duty, there is no legal responsibility to act even though an EMT-I may feel a moral obligation to help.

46. **The answer is B.** (Mosby, *Medical/Legal Considerations.* Brady, *Medical-Legal Considerations of Emergency Care.*) (A), (C), and (D) are correct. (B) is incorrect because the act or omission must have been below, not above, the standard of care.

47. **Answers.** (Brady, *Medical-Legal Considerations of Emergency Care.*)
   (A) 2
   (B) 4
   (C) 3
   (D) 1

48. **The answer is C.** (Mosby, *Medical/Legal Considerations.*) (A), (B), and (D) are parts of the process of obtaining informed consent. (C) is incorrect because providing exact doses and references is not appropriate or required in obtaining informed consent.

49. **Answers.** (Mosby, *Medical/Legal Considerations.*)
   (A) 6
   (B) 4
   (C) 3
   (D) 1
   (E) 2
   (F) 5

50. **The answer is A.** (Mosby, *Medical/Legal Considerations.*) The patients described in (B), (C), and (D) are frequently subjected to the use of force and restraint. (A) is incorrect because it is not permissible to force or restrain a patient merely because that patient is verbally abusive to the EMT-I.

51. **The answer is D.** (Mosby, *Medical/Legal Considerations.*) (D) is correct because the state law would provide guidelines on the use of force and restraint of a patient. (A), (B), and (C) are all incorrect.

52. The answer is C. (Mosby, *Medical/Legal Considerations.*) (A), (B), and (D) are all correct. (C) is incorrect because COBRA stands for the Consolidated Omnibus Budget Reconciliation Act of 1985.

53. The answer is C. (Mosby, *Medical/Legal Considerations.*) (A), (B), and (D) are correct. (C) is incorrect because inventory checklists may be helped by chart documentation but do not carry the same importance to the patient and/or from a medical-legal standpoint.

EMS
COMMUNICATIONS

In this chapter, you will review:

- digital coders and repeater/nonrepeater systems

- role of the EMS dispatcher

- proper radio transmission

EMS COMMUNICATIONS

Directions: Each item below contains four suggested responses. Select the **one best** response to each item.

54. Match each of the components of an emergency medical system (EMS) communication with the correct function:

(A) Base station _____
(B) Mobile radios _____
(C) Dedicated landlines _____
(D) Cellular telephones _____
(E) Portable radios _____
(F) Enhanced 911 _____

1. Mounted two-way radios
2. Access number for EMS
3. Site with most powerful radio in EMS system
4. Hand-held devices that allow EMT-Is to communicate away from an ambulance
5. Rapid means of communication between the public and EMS providers
6. EMS dispatchers' telephone lines to EMS personnel, hospitals, police, fire department, etc.

55. Which of the following is an advantage of a repeater over a nonrepeater system?

(A) All communications are repeated twice in case there is a questionable message
(B) Repeats messages only from EMS prehospital providers
(C) Allows two messages to be sent at the same time over the same frequency
(D) Receives a transmission from a low-power portable or mobile radio on one frequency, and then transmits at higher power on another frequency

56. Which of the following BEST explains the proper use of a digital encoder?

(A) It allows labeling of sensitive EMS equipment

(B) It allows rapid identification of EMS personnel

(C) It is a telephone keypad-size device that generates unique codes or tones recognized by another radio's decoder

(D) It is a cellular phone device that allows base stations to recognize certain EMT-I transmissions

57. All of the following are the functions and responsibilities of the Federal Communications Commission (FCC) EXCEPT

(A) licensing and allocating radio frequencies

(B) spot-checking base stations and dispatch centers for licenses and records

(C) selling state-of-the-art communications equipment and supplies

(D) monitoring radio frequencies for appropriate usage

58. All of the following are phases of communications involved in completing an EMS event EXCEPT

(A) a telephone request for help via 911

(B) an emergency medical dispatcher's notification to an available EMS crew

(C) an EMT-I's notification of his or her run times, including en route to scene time, on the scene time, en route to hospital time, hospital arrival time, in-service time, and off the air time

(D) an EMT-I's personal communications with his or her family concerning his or her arrival home time

59. All of the following are responsibilities of EMS dispatchers EXCEPT

(A) limiting a 911 caller's information to name, location, and nature of call

(B) directing the appropriate EMS unit to respond to a call

(C) ensuring the safety of all EMS responders

(D) maintaining written records of the call

60. All of the following are pieces of information which a dispatcher must attempt to obtain from a caller EXCEPT

(A) location and nature of the emergency

(B) call-back number for the caller

(C) insurance coverage and policy numbers

(D) additional specific information to help determine the severity and nature of the emergency

61. All of the following are reasons for an EMT-I to provide verbal communication of patient information to the hospital EXCEPT

  (A) to obtain advice on how to encourage a patient with altered mental status to sign a refusal of medical care form

  (B) to obtain orders for prehospital care

  (C) to assist the hospital in preparing for the arrival of an emergently ill patient

  (D) to assist with resolving uncertainty about continuing or terminating a resuscitation

62. Arrange the following patient assessment information in the correct order for radio transmission to the physician:

  (A) EMT-I's identification number and level of training of provider _____

  (B) Estimated time of arrival at hospital _____

  (C) Pertinent past medical history, medications, and allergies _____

  (D) Physical examination findings _____

  (E) Scene description _____

  (F) Orders being requested _____

  (G) Treatment given so far _____

  (H) Response to treatment _____

  (I) Name of private physician _____

  (J) Patient's age and sex _____

  (K) Brief description of present illness _____

  (L) Chief complaint _____

63. All of the following are important communication techniques which influence the clarity of radio transmission EXCEPT

  (A) be jovial and entertaining

  (B) be clear

  (C) be concise

  (D) be professional

64. All of the following techniques are used to properly receive and transmit information on mobile and portable radios EXCEPT

  (A) before transmitting, listening to the frequency to make sure no one else is transmitting

  (B) making sure the unit being called signals that it is ready to receive the transmission

  (C) using abbreviations and codes to save time

  (D) after receiving orders from a physician, repeating them back to the physician

65. Which of the following positions of a portable radio's antenna provides maximum coverage?

  (A) Horizontal

  (B) Inverted (upside down)

  (C) Vertical (upright)

  (D) Diagonal

EMS COMMUNICATIONS

54. Answers. (Mosby, *EMS Communications.* Brady, *EMS Communications.*)
- (A) 3
- (B) 1
- (C) 6
- (D) 5
- (E) 4
- (F) 2

55. The answer is D. (Mosby, *EMS Communications.* Brady, *EMS Communications.*) (D) is correct. (A) and (B) are incorrect because a repeater does not duplicate messages. (C) is incorrect because a repeater is not capable of transmitting two messages at the same time.

56. The answer is C. (Brady, *EMS Communications.*) (C) is correct. Each base station has a decoder which recognizes only its own tone or a code sent by the encoder. This activates the base station's receiving capability. (A), (B), and (D) are all incorrect.

57. The answer is C. (Brady, *EMS Communications.*) (A), (B), (D), establishing technical standards for radio equipment and licensing and regulating the personnel who repair and operate radio equipment are some of the functions and responsibilities of the FCC. (C) is incorrect because the FCC is not involved in the selling of communications equipment or supplies.

58. The answer is D. (Mosby, *EMS Communications.*) (A), (B), and (C) and medical communications are some of the phases of the communications involved in completing an EMS event. (D) is incorrect because an EMT-I's personal communications with his or her family have nothing to do with an EMS event.

59. The answer is A. (Brady, *EMS Communications.* Mosby, *EMS Communications.*) (B), (C), (D), providing prearrival instructions to the caller until emergency care arrives, monitoring communications among EMS and other public safety personnel, and resolving any communication difficulties are some of the responsibilities of an EMS dispatcher. (A) is incorrect because a dispatcher should try to obtain as much information as possible about the emergency from the caller.

60. The answer is C. (Brady, *EMS Communications.* Mosby, *EMS Communications.*) (A), (B), and (D) are key pieces of information needed from each caller. (C) is incorrect because this is inappropriate information for a dispatcher to request. It only delays the dispatching of the correct EMS providers and the handling of other emergent calls.

61. The answer is A. (Mosby, *EMS Communications.*) (B), (C), (D), soliciting advice on the treatment of a patient with an uncertain problem, requesting a physician's assistance to encourage an obviously sick patient to accept care and/or transport to the hospital, resolving difficulties with non-EMS physicians interfering with the care of the patient, and reviewing the situation when transport appears to be unnecessary, are all responsibilities of an EMT-I. (A) is incorrect becaue the EMT-I must never encourage a patient with an altered mental status to sign a refusal of medical care form. The altered mental status patient may have a life-threatening underlying medical condition which is causing his or her condition, for example, acute cerebrovascular accident, drug overdose, hypoxia, etc.

62. Answers. (Mosby, *EMS Communications.*)
A, E, J, L, K, C, D, G, H, F, I, B

63. The answer is A. (Mosby, *EMS Communications.*) (B), (C), and (D) are correct. (A) is incorrect because there is no need to provide entertainment during the communication of important and often critical patient care information.

64. The answer is C. (Mosby, *EMS Communications.*) (A), (B), and (D) are correct. (C) is incorrect because one usually should try to avoid the use of codes and abbreviations unless they are a regular part of the system.

65. The answer is C. (Mosby, *EMS Communications.*) (C) is the correct position. (A), (B), and (D) all describe incorrect positions.

DOCUMENTATION

In this chapter, you will review:

- reasons for patient care documentation

- key components of the written report

- special documentation considerations

DOCUMENTATION

Directions: Each item below contains four suggested responses. Select the **one best** response to each item.

66. All of the following are reasons to perform patient care documentation EXCEPT

    (A) to provide an inventory of drugs and supplies

    (B) to provide a record of the pre-hospital treatment administered

    (C) to allow medical direction to perform quality improvement audits and document the following of protocols

    (D) to provide otherwise unobtainable information to the hospital staff, such as vehicle damage from a motor vehicle accident

67. All of the following are reasons why an emergency medical system needs to gather data from run reports EXCEPT

    (A) to release patient care information to the press immediately

    (B) to provide information for quality assurance and continuing improvement of the system

    (C) to assist with revenue collections and operational statistics

    (D) to help identify EMT-Intermediates (EMT-Is) who may require additional training and skill practice

68. All of the following are components of the written report and the information which should be included in it EXCEPT

(A) dispatch information: includes address, type of call, priority level, dispatch time, and call number

(B) chief complaint: a listing of the medical problem which prompted the patient or any other person to call for an ambulance

(C) important observations: particularly of the scene with regard to the mechanism of injury, the use of safety equipment, reasons for refusing treatment

(D) verbal disagreements with one's partner concerning the best route for transporting a patient to the hospital

69. All of the following are pieces of information that should be included in the written report EXCEPT

(A) present illness, including time of onset, location, frequency, quality, character of the problem, setting, alleviating factors, and aggravating factors

(B) past medical history, including hospitalizations, surgeries, injuries, illnesses, allergies, medications, and patient's physician

(C) physical assessment, including vital signs (repeated as necessary), condition of patient on arrival, pertinent physical findings

(D) details of patient's last normal physical examination performed in the patient's doctor's office

70. The EMT-I documenting the patient care record notices that he or she has made a mistake on the written record. Which of the following is the proper way to correct the mistake?

(A) Destroy the record and begin a new chart

(B) Draw a single horizontal line through the incorrect entry so that it remains legible

(C) White out the mistake and write over it

(D) Use a black magic marker to cover over the mistake and start again

71. The EMT-I is confronted with a 50-year-old male who is complaining of abdominal pain. After a focused history and physical examination, the patient adamantly refuses to go to the hospital. All of the following are parts of the correct approach to dealing with a patient who refuses care EXCEPT

(A) making a clear effort to persuade the patient to go to the hospital

(B) respecting the patient's right to refuse care immediately even if the patient has an altered mental status from illness, alcohol, drugs, etc.

(C) if the patient can make a rational, competent decision, getting the patient's signature to document the refusal of care

(D) if the patient refuses to sign the refusal form, having a police officer, bystander, or family member sign the form along with his or her printed name, address, and telephone number

DOCUMENTATION

ANSWERS

66. The answer is A. (Mosby, *Medical Terminology.*) (B), (C), and (D) are correct. (A) is incorrect because supply inventories are part of operations, not of patient care documentation.

67. The answer is A. (Mosby, *Documentation.*) (B), (C), (D), assisting with training program development and research are some of the reasons for gathering data from run reports. (A) is incorrect because patient care information is confidential and can be released only after a patient has given permission.

68. The answer is D. (Mosby, *Documentation.*) (A), (B), and (C) are correct. (D) is incorrect because the written report is not the place to report personal interactions that are not related to the care of the patient.

69. The answer is D. (Mosby, *Documentation.*) (A), (B), (C), treatments provided, response to treatment, demographic information, billing information, actual run times, run disposition, and signatures are all parts of the written record. (D) is incorrect because the full details of a patient's last physical examination are superfluous. However, noting a particular facet of the last examination that is related to the problem at hand may be helpful.

70. The answer is B. (Mosby, *Documentation.*) (B) is correct. After this is done, the correct information should be added. The EMT-I may choose to describe the reason for the correction and/or have it witnessed. (A), (C), and (D) are all incorrect.

71. The answer is B. (Mosby, *Documentation.*) (A), (C), and (D) are all correct. (B) is incorrect because patients with altered mental status should never be asked to sign a refusal of care form.

MEDICAL
TERMINOLOGY

In this chapter, you will review:

- common word roots, prefixes and suffixes

- common medical abbreviations

- body movement descriptions

MEDICAL TERMINOLOGY

Directions: Each item below contains four suggested responses. Select the **one best** response to each item.

72. Medical terminology is BEST defined as

(A) the language used in an operating room

(B) a special vocabulary used in the medical field

(C) a language used only by insurance companies dealing with medical claims

(D) a language consisting only of medical abbreviations

73. All of the following are word roots EXCEPT

(A) *abdomino*

(B) *derm*

(C) *tachy*

(D) *post*

74. All of the following are prefixes EXCEPT

(A) *ab*

(B) *emia*

(C) *erythro*

(D) *patho*

75. All of the following are suffixes EXCEPT

(A) *semi*

(B) *scopy*

(C) *uria*

(D) *ectomy*

76. All of the following are combining forms EXCEPT

(A) *gastro-*

(B) *cardio-*

(C) *cysto-*

(D) *hypo*

77. All of the following are combining forms EXCEPT

(A) *thyro-*
(B) *vaso-*
(C) *tracheo-*
(D) *center*

78. A combining vowel is a vowel which is added to a word root before a suffix. All of the following provide examples of the use of a combining vowel EXCEPT

(A) *uretero*
(B) *viscero*
(C) *brachio*
(D) *solo*

79. All of the following are planes of the human body EXCEPT

(A) sagittal
(B) horizontal
(C) frontal
(D) transverse

80. Match each directional term with the correct definition:

(A) Inferior _____
(B) Cranial _____
(C) Posterior _____
(D) Medial _____
(E) Proximal _____
(F) Caudal _____
(G) Superior _____
(H) Lateral _____
(I) Anterior _____
(J) Distal _____

1. Nearest the origin of a structure
2. In or near the head
3. Below or lower
4. Toward the front or belly
5. Toward the back
6. Toward the midline
7. Near sacrum of spinal column
8. Above or higher
9. Away from midline
10. Farthest from origin of a structure

81. Match each body movement with the correct definition:

(A) Abduction _____
(B) Flexion _____
(C) Rotation _____
(D) Adduction _____
(E) Circumduction _____
(F) Extension _____

1. Decreases a joint angle, bringing the parts together
2. Swinging of a body part in a circle
3. Moving away from the midline
4. Increases a joint angle, bringing the parts farther apart
5. Moving toward the midline
6. Twisting or turning apart on its axis

82. All of the following are correct definitions of body postures EXCEPT

(A) erect: standing in an upright
position
(B) supine: lying on the back with the
face up
(C) prone: lying on the stomach with
the face down
(D) sideward: lying on the right or
left side

MEDICAL TERMINOLOGY

ANSWERS

72. The answer is B. (Mosby, *Medical Terminology.*) (B) is correct. (A), (C), and (D) refer to locations or situations where medical terminology is used.

73. The answer is D. (Brady, *Medical Terminology.*) (A), (B), and (C) are word roots which determine the essential meaning of a word. (D) is incorrect because *post* is a prefix, not a word root.

74. The answer is B. (Brady, *Medical Terminology.*) (A), (C), and (D) are all prefixes. *Ab* means "away" (e.g., *abnormal*), *erythro* means "red" (e.g., *erythrocyte*), and *patho* means "disease" (e.g., *pathophysiology*). (B) is incorrect because *emia* is a suffix meaning "related to the blood."

75. The answer is A. (Brady, *Medical Terminology.*) (B), (C), and (D) are all suffixes. *Scopy* means "examination with an instrument" (e.g., *colonoscopy*), *uria* means "related to the urine" (e.g., *hematuria*), and *ectomy* means "cutting out" (e.g., *lumpectomy*). (A) is incorrect because *semi* is a prefix meaning "half."

76. The answer is D. (Mosby, *Medical Terminology.*) (A), (B), and (C) are all combining forms. A combining form is used to join a word root with a vowel and is followed by a hyphen. *Gastro* means "stomach" (e.g., gastromegaly), *cardio* means "heart" (e.g., cardiology), and *cysto* means "bladder" (e.g., cystoscopy). (D) is incorrect because *hypo* is a prefix meaning "under" or "deficient." It is not followed by a hyphen.

77. The answer is D. (Mosby, *Medical Terminology.*) A combining form is a word root with an added vowel. *Thyro* stands for "thyroid," *vas* stands for "vessel," and *tracheo* stands for "trachea." (D) is incorrect because *center* is a word which stands only for itself. It is not a combining form.

78. The answer is D. (Mosby, *Medical Terminology.*) (A), (B), and (C) are all correct examples. (D) is incorrect because *solo* is a word which does not contain a combining vowel.

79. The answer is B. (Mosby, *Medical Terminology.*) Sagittal, frontal, transverse, and midsagittal are the four planes of the human body. (B) is incorrect because there is no such body plane as the horizontal.

80. Answers (Mosby, *Medical Terminology.*)
(A) 3
(B) 2
(C) 5
(D) 6
(E) 1
(F) 7
(G) 8
(H) 9
(I) 4
(J) 10

81. Answers (Mosby, *Medical Terminology.*)
(A) 3
(B) 1
(C) 6
(D) 5
(E) 2
(F) 4

82. The answer is D. (Mosby, *Medical Terminology.*) (A), (B), and (C) and the lateral recumbent posture are the four body postures. (D) is incorrect because sideward is not a body posture. Actually, the lateral recumbent posture involves lying on the right or left side.

BODY SYSTEMS

In this chapter, you will review:

- structure of the major organ systems
- functions of the major organ systems

BODY SYSTEMS

Directions: Each item below contains four suggested responses. Select the **one best** response to each item.

83. Which of the following is the correct definition of *connective tissue*?

(A) Connects tendons to muscles
(B) Links cardiac conduction systems to cardiac muscle
(C) Binds other types of tissue together
(D) Connects lung alveoli to pericardium

84. All of the following are body cavities EXCEPT

(A) thoracic cavity
(B) cranial cavity
(C) urinary cavity
(D) spinal cavity

85. Match each medical term with the correct definition:

(A) Cartilage _____
(B) Tendon _____
(C) Ligament _____
(D) Joint _____

1. Fibrous tissue which attaches bone to cartilage
2. White fibrous tissue which attaches muscle to bone
3. Site where two or more bones meet or articulate
4. Connective tissue found primarily in joints

86. Which of the following are the names of the two major divisions of the skeletal system?

(A) Skull and vertebrae
(B) Axial skeleton and vertebrae
(C) Skull and long bones
(D) Axial skeleton and appendicular skeleton

87. Which of the following is the BEST definition of the structure and function of the muscular system?

    (A) Composed of contractile tissues which are responsible for movement

    (B) A network of muscles which contract and relax

    (C) Extremities linked to the body which act independently

    (D) Made up of individual joints which are responsible for walking

88. All of the following are types of muscle EXCEPT

    (A) skeletal

    (B) circular

    (C) cardiac

    (D) smooth

89. All of the following are parts of the structure of the circulatory system EXCEPT

    (A) heart

    (B) blood vessels

    (C) blood

    (D) kidneys

90. Match the following structures of the circulatory system with the correct functions:

    (A) Heart _____

    (B) Red blood cells _____

    (C) Arteries _____

    (D) Platelets _____

    (E) Veins _____

    (F) White blood cells _____

    (G) Blood _____

    1. Help the body fight infections

    2. Carry blood away from the heart

    3. Pumps blood throughout the body

    4. Return deoxygenated blood back to the heart

    5. Contain hemoglobin and deliver oxygen to tissues

    6. Clump together to assist blood clotting

    7. Fluid tissue consisting of cells and plasma

91. The respiratory system can BEST be defined as the body system which

    (A) allows the exchange of oxygen and carbon dioxide in blood

    (B) inspires and expires air

    (C) produces sputum and wheezing

    (D) maintains the airway and cough reflex

92. All of the following are parts of the structure of the respiratory system EXCEPT

    (A) mouth

    (B) oral and nasal cavities

    (C) bronchi

    (D) sinuses

93. Which of the following is the BEST definition of the function of the nervous system?

(A) Conducts information only for involuntary actions
(B) Produces a state of continuous anxiety in the body
(C) Conducts information that controls and coordinates the body
(D) Primarily controls the sensory messages which the extremities pick up

94. All of the following are parts of the structure of the nervous system EXCEPT

(A) brain
(B) spinal nerves
(C) autonomic nervous system
(D) vertebrae

95. All of the following are true statements about the autonomic nervous system EXCEPT

(A) it controls the voluntary functions of the nervous system
(B) the sympathetic branch controls the constriction of blood vessels, increases in heart rate and blood pressure, and a feeling of nervousness in a stressful situation
(C) the parasympathetic branch is responsible for increasing the heart rate, intestinal activity, the respiratory rate, and pupillary reactions
(D) it is a part of the peripheral nervous system

96. Match the four quadrants of the abdomen with the correct contents of each quadrant:

(A) Right upper quadrant _____
(B) Left upper quadrant _____
(C) Left lower quadrant _____
(D) Right lower quadrant _____

1. Appendix, right ovary, right ureter, uterus, urinary bladder, part of right colon
2. Gallbladder, liver, right kidney, part of right and transverse colon
3. Part of left colon, left ureter, left ovary, uterus, urinary bladder
4. Part of left and transverse colon, left kidney, spleen, stomach, pancreas

97. The BEST description of the function of the urinary system is that it

(A) provides an area for disposal of excess water
(B) provides a link to the genital system in males
(C) provides a means of excreting the bacteria related to a urinary infection
(D) provides a means for the removal of waste products from the body

98. All of the following are parts of the structure of the urinary system EXCEPT

(A) gallbladder
(B) kidneys
(C) ureters
(D) urethra

99. Which of the following BEST describes the function of the reproductive system?

(A) Removal of bodily wastes
(B) Pleasure center
(C) Sexual reproduction
(D) Storage of genetic material

100. The structure of the male reproductive system includes all of the following EXCEPT

    (A) penis
    (B) prostate
    (C) testicles
    (D) urinary bladder

101. The female reproductive system includes all of the following EXCEPT

    (A) urethra
    (B) vagina
    (C) uterus
    (D) ovary

102. Which of the following BEST describes the function of the immune system?

    (A) provides the body with a series of antibodies
    (B) provides the body with protection against AIDS
    (C) protects the body from foreign materials
    (D) protects the body from thermal injury

103. The immune system is made up of two types of immunity. Which of the following include these two types?

    (A) General and specific
    (B) Individual and herd immunity
    (C) Specific and nonspecific immunity
    (D) Autoimmune and individual immunity

104. All of the following are ductless glands, which are part of the endocrine system, EXCEPT

    (A) thyroid and pituitary
    (B) ovaries and testes
    (C) salivary and sweat glands
    (D) adrenals and pancreas

105. Match each of the following glands with its correct function:

    (A) Thyroid _____
    (B) Parathyroids _____
    (C) Ovaries _____
    (D) Pituitary _____
    (E) Pancreas _____
    (F) Testes _____
    (G) Adrenals _____

    1. Cause facial hair, deep voice, and reproductive changes in males
    2. Produces insulin and glucagon and digestive enzymes
    3. Produce sex hormones, epinephrine, and norepinephrine
    4. Secretes hormones which regulate growth metabolism
    5. Produce hormones which maintain blood calcium levels
    6. Produce hormones which cause breast development and female reproductive changes
    7. Produces hormones which regulate the functions of other endocrine glands

BODY SYSTEMS

A N S W E R S

83. The answer is C. (Mosby, *Body Systems.*) (C) is correct. Examples of connective tissue are bone, cartilage, and fat. (A), (B), and (D) are all incorrect definitions.

84. The answer is C. (Mosby, *Body Systems.*) The thoracic cavity, cranial cavity, spinal cavity, abdominal cavity, and pelvic cavity are the five body cavities. (C) is incorrect because although there is a urinary system, it is not called a cavity.

85. Answers. (Mosby, *Body Systems.*)
   (A) 4
   (B) 2
   (C) 1
   (D) 3

86. The answer is D. (Mosby, *Body Systems.*) (A), (B), and (C) are incorrect. (D) is correct. The axial skeleton consists of the entire torso, including the skull (which surrounds the brain), the spine (which provides the primary support of the body), the ribs (which protect the thoracic cavity), and the sternum. The appendicular skeleton consists of the four extremities, the shoulder girdle (which attaches the upper extremities to the body), and the pelvic girdle (which attaches the lower extremities to the body).

87. The answer is A. (Mosby, *Body Systems.*) (A) is correct. (B) is incorrect because while the structure of the muscular system could be defined as a network of muscles, its function involves more than simply contraction and relaxation. (C) and (D) are incorrect because the structure of the muscular system does not consist of extremities or joints.

88. The answer is B. (Mosby, *Body Systems.*) (A), (C), and (D) are correct. (B) is incorrect because there is no circular type of muscle.

89. The answer is D. (Mosby, *Body Systems.*) (A), (B), and (C) make up the circulatory system of the body. (D) is incorrect because the kidneys are part of the urinary system, not the circulatory system.

90. Answers. (Mosby, *Body Systems.*)
   (A) 3
   (B) 5
   (C) 2
   (D 6
   (E) 4
   (F) 1
   (G) 7

91. The answer is A. (Mosby, *Body Systems.*) (A) defines the correct function of the respiratory system. (B), (C), and (D) are all incorrect as definitions of the respiratory system.

92. The answer is D. (Mosby, *Body Systems.*) (A), (B), (C), the larynx, vocal cords, the trachea, the bronchioles, and the alveoli are all parts of the structure of the respiratory system. The respiratory system is often divided into the upper and lower systems. The upper system consists of the mouth, nasal and oral cavities, larynx, and vocal cords. The lower system consists of the trachea, bronchi, bronchioles, and alveoli. (D) is incorrect because the sinuses, despite being frequently affected by the respiratory system, are not considered part of the respiratory system.

93. The answer is C. (Mosby, *Body Systems.*) (C) is correct. (A), (B), and (D) are incorrect definitions because each describes only one of the functions of the nervous system.

94. The answer is D. (Mosby, *Body Systems.*) (A), (B), and (C), the spinal cord, and the cranial nerves are all parts of the nervous system. (D) is incorrect because even though the vertebrae surround the spinal cord, they are not considered part of the nervous system.

95. The answer is C. (Mosby, *Body Systems.*) (A), (B), and (D) are all correct. (C) is incorrect because the parasympathetic nervous system is responsible for slowing the heart rate, intestinal activity, the respiratory rate, and pupillary reactions.

96. Answers. (Mosby, *Body Systems.*)
   (A) 2
   (B) 4
   (C) 3
   (D) 1

97. The answer is D. (Mosby, *Body Systems.*) (D) is correct. The urinary system also helps maintain a balance of salt and water in the body. (A), (B), and (C) are incorrect because while each may describe an activity of the urinary system, it is not the best description of the system's function.

98. The answer is A. (Mosby, *Body Systems.*) The kidneys, ureters, urethra, and urinary bladder are parts of the structure of the urinary system. (A) is incorrect because the urinary bladder not the gallbladder, is part of the urinary system.

99. The answer is C. (Mosby, *Body Systems.*) (C) is the correct answer despite popular opinion. (A), (B), and (D) are incorrect descriptions.

100. The answer is D. (Mosby, *Body Systems.*) The penis, prostate, testicles, seminal vesicles, and urethra are all parts of the structure of the male reproductive system. (D) is incorrect because the urinary bladder is part of the urinary system.

101. The answer is A. (Mosby, *Body Systems.*) The vagina, uterus, ovaries, fallopian tubes, and cervix are all parts of the female reproductive system. (A) is incorrect because in a female the urethra is only a part of the urinary system. By contrast, in a male the urethra is a part of both the urinary and the reproductive systems.

102. The answer is C. (Mosby, *Body Systems.*) (C) is correct. (A) and (B) are incorrect because these are only aspects of the function of the immune system. (D) is incorrect because the immune system is not involved in the body's response to thermal injury.

103. The answer is C. (Mosby, *Body Systems.*) (C) is the correct answer. Nonspecific immunity involves three mechanisms: mechanical barriers (such as the skin), chemical barriers (such as histamine release), and white blood cells that ingest and destroy bacteria and foreign bodies. Two types of specific immunity exist: antibody production to a given antigen and cell-mediated immunity through the action of lymphocytes. (A), (B), and (D) are all incorrect.

104. The answer is C. (Mosby, *Body Systems.*) (A), (B), and (D), the pineal, the hypothalamus, the thymus, and the parathyroids are ductless glands and are parts of the endocrine system. (C) is incorrect because these glands are not related to the endocrine system.

105. Answers. (Mosby, *Body Systems.*)
 (A) 4
 (B) 5
 (C) 6
 (D) 7
 (E) 2
 (F) 1
 (G) 3

PATIENT ASSESSMENT AND INITIAL MANAGEMENT

In this chapter, you will review:

- phases of physical assessment

- body substance isolation precautions

- initial, focused, detailed and ongoing assessment

PATIENT ASSESSMENT AND INITIAL MANAGEMENT

Directions: Each item below contains four suggested responses. Select the **one best** response to each item.

106. All of the following are phases of the physical assessment performed by an EMT-Intermediate (EMT-I) EXCEPT

(A) sizing up the scene
(B) initial assessment
(C) resuscitation
(D) telemetry communication

107. All of the following are examples of potential scene hazards which may endanger an EMT-I or patient EXCEPT

(A) an elderly patient
(B) a hazardous materials spill
(C) extreme heights
(D) a violent patient

108. All of the following are parts of the initial assessment of an emergently ill patient EXCEPT

(A) general impression and mechanism of injury
(B) assessment of mental status (AVPU)
(C) application of pulse oximetry
(D) accessing the airway

109. After arriving at the scene of a motor vehicle accident, an EMT-I begins to perform an initial assessment. All of the following are parts of the mechanism of the injury/nature of the illness which can affect the emergent care of a patient EXCEPT

(A) obtaining a family history and an immunization history

(B) a surviving occupant of the car notes that the driver of the car passed out before the accident

(C) assessing the location and the amount of damage to the car

(D) rapid triage and assessment of all victims

110. The AVPU method of evaluating a patient's level of responsiveness includes all of the following EXCEPT

(A) A = awake and alert

(B) V = patient responds to verbal stimuli

(C) P = patient responds to painful stimuli

(D) U = patient is unstable

111. The most important indication for providing cervical spine immobilization is

(A) any patient with loss of consciousness

(B) a cervical spine injury is present or suspected

(C) isolated extremity trauma

(D) arthritis of the cervical spine

112. All of the following are methods of providing cervical spine immobilization EXCEPT

(A) an EMT-I providing manual immobilization

(B) applying a rigid extrication collar

(C) if a rigid collar is not available, having the EMT-I stabilize the head between his or her knees

(D) using a soft cervical collar

113. All of the following are techniques for evaluating the effectiveness of ventilation EXCEPT

(A) chest wall rise

(B) skin temperature

(C) normalization of heart rate

(D) auscultation of lungs

114. You respond to the scene of a "stabbing" and find a 22-year-old male lying in a pool of blood, lethargic and very pale. Your partner confirms an open airway and adequate ventilation and then asks you to assess the patient's circulation. All of the following are parts of the mechanism for evaluating the effectiveness of perfusion EXCEPT

(A) assessing the patient's pulses

(B) checking the patient's pulse rate

(C) checking capillary refill in adults only, not in infants and children

(D) checking skin color, moisture, and temperature

115. Each of the following palpable pulses represents an estimate of systolic blood pressure EXCEPT

(A) carotid, 60 mm Hg systolic
(B) femoral, 70 mm Hg systolic
(C) radial, 80 mm Hg systolic
(D) aorta, 120 mm Hg systolic

116. In trying to identify "priority" patients, which of the following is the BEST definition?

(A) Unstable patients who require an advanced level of care as soon as possible
(B) VIP patients
(C) Stable patients who want to be taken to the hospital immediately
(D) Stable patients who have the potential to become unstable

117. All of the following are examples of priority patients EXCEPT

(A) responsive with stable vital signs, difficulty breathing, childbirth
(B) shock, unresponsive, failure to correct hypoxia
(C) severe hypertension, complicated childbirth, severe pain
(D) chest pain with systolic blood pressure less than 100, uncontrolled bleeding, multiple trauma

118. Medical control has provided EMT-Is with various approaches to treating priority patients. Some of the possible options include the following EXCEPT

(A) rapid transport to the nearest medical facility
(B) activating an aeromedical helicopter service
(C) a high-speed ambulance ride with lights and sirens for all priority patients
(D) requesting immediate advanced life support (ALS) care by paramedics

119. All of the following are parts of the focused assessment for a trauma patient EXCEPT

(A) reconsidering the mechanism of injury and the transport decision
(B) completing the rapid assessment of the ABCDEs; (A) airway, (B) breathing, (C) circulation, (D) disability, (E) exposure
(C) performing rapid trauma assessment
(D) beginning two large-bore intravenous lines of Ringer's lactate and normal saline

120. In performing a focused assessment of a trauma patient's vital signs, it is important to remember the normal ranges for blood pressure. All of the following are correct EXCEPT

(A) newborn, 70/40 mm Hg
(B) up to 1 year of age, 86/60 mm Hg
(C) over 2 years of age, lower limit of systolic blood pressure is 70 plus 10 times the age in years
(D) adult, 80–110 mm Hg systolic and 40–60 mm Hg diastolic

121. You are dispatched to an elderly male who fell down a full flight of stairs. As you arrive at the scene, you are directed to the basement. You find an 88-year-old male who is unconscious and has a large scalp laceration. Your first priority is to

(A) start a large-bore intravenous line with lactated Ringer's
(B) begin to take a set of vital signs
(C) assess for the amount of neurologic disability
(D) with cervical spine precautions, establish an airway with the jaw thrust maneuver

122. All of the following are the normal respiratory rates in the listed age groups EXCEPT

(A) newborn, 25 breaths per minute
(B) infant (less than 1 year of age), 20–30 breaths per minute
(C) child, 18–26 breaths per minute
(D) adult, 12–20 breaths per minute

123. The following are the normal pulse rates for the listed age groups EXCEPT

(A) newborn to 3 years, 100–160 beats per minute
(B) child (3 to 8 years), 70–150 beats per minute
(C) older child (8 to 12 years), 55–150 beats per minute
(D) adolescent (over 12 years), 60–110 beats per minute

124. All of the following are parts of the focused assessment of an unresponsive medical (nontraumatic) emergently ill patient EXCEPT

(A) rapid airway assessment
(B) a complete SAMPLE history
(C) administering intravenous narcan
(D) taking a set of baseline vital signs

125. In performing a focused assessment of a responsive medical (nontraumatic) emergently ill patient, it is often helpful to use the OPQRST acronym. These letters stand for

O = _____
P = _____
Q = _____
R = _____
S = _____
T = _____

126. All of the following are parts of the detailed assessment of a patient EXCEPT

(A) chief complaint
(B) patient history
(C) second and third sets of vital signs
(D) head-to-toe examination

127. Which of the following patient scenarios would call for the performance of a detailed assessment on the scene?

(A) A fingertip laceration
(B) A cardiac arrest victim failing to respond to defibrillation and cardiopulmonary resuscitation (CPR)
(C) A patient with massive gastrointestinal bleeding that is worsening despite vigorous intravenous fluid resuscitation and a pneumatic antishock garment
(D) A responsive 76-year-old man who has fallen down a flight of stairs and has a probable hip fracture and stable vital signs.

128. In performing the neurologic part of the head-to-toe examination, the use of the Glasgow Coma Scale has been found to be particularly helpful in assessing trauma patients. All of the following are correct statements concerning this scale EXCEPT

(A) the maximum score is 15 and the minimum is 3
(B) the range of the best motor response is 6 to 1
(C) the range of the best verbal response is 5 to 1
(D) the range of eye opening is 5 to 1

129. Providing an ongoing assessment of a patient includes all of the following parameters EXCEPT

(A) monitoring the airway, breathing, and skin color, temperature, and condition
(B) reassessing mental status, pulse, and vital signs
(C) contacting medical control, discussing the case with one's partner, and reviewing protocols
(D) realigning patient priorities, repeating focused examinations, and checking efficacy of treatment and interventions

130. Which of the following are the correct time intervals for an EMT-I performing an ongoing assessment?

(A) Stable patients every 20 minutes, unstable patients every 10 minutes
(B) Stable patients every 30 minutes, unstable patients every 15 minutes
(C) Stable patients every 25 minutes, unstable patients every 10 minutes, cardiac arrest patients every 2 minutes
(D) Stable patients every 15 minutes, unstable patients every 5 minutes

131. All of the following are factors which help determine the facility to which a patient is transported EXCEPT

(A) patient's condition
(B) available facilities
(C) available copies of medical records
(D) available transportation modalities

132. In transporting a patient, it is very important to contact medical control or the receiving facility to relay all of the following information EXCEPT

(A) the patient's next of kin
(B) the nature of the incident
(C) life-threatening problems
(D) the estimated time of arrival

133. All of the following are benefits of providing accurate documentation of patient care EXCEPT that it

(A) provides a clear and readable record of the patient care rendered
(B) permits an EMT-I to go beyond the scope of practice
(C) facilitates transfer of the patient to the receiving facility
(D) assists in justification of patient care in judicial hearings

PATIENT ASSESSMENT AND INITIAL MANAGEMENT

ANSWERS

106. **The answer is D.** (Mosby, *Patient Assessment.*) (A), (B), (C), a focused history and physical examination, a detailed assessment, and ongoing field management are the six phases of physical assessment by an EMT-I. (D) is incorrect because telemetry communication is not related to the phases of physical assessment.

107. **The answer is A.** (Brady, *General Patient Assessment and Initial Management.*) A hazardous materials spill, extreme heights, and violent patient, and water hazards, biological hazards, bloodborne pathogens, and electrical wires are some of the potential hazards an EMT-I may encounter. (A) is incorrect because an elderly patient does not constitute a scene hazard.

108. **The answer is C.** (Mosby, *Patient Assessment.*) (A), (B), (D), assessment of breathing, assessment of circulation, and the identification of unstable patients are parts of the initial assessment. (C) is an adjunct to the assessment of an emergently ill patient but is not a key part of the initial assessment.

109. **The answer is A.** (Mosby, *Patient Assessment.*) (B), (C), and (D) are parts of the initial assessment. (A) is not related to the mechanism of the injury and/or the nature of the illness.

110. **The answer is D.** (Mosby, *Patient Assessment.*) (A), (B), and (C) are correct. (D) is incorrect because U = patient is unresponsive.

111. **The answer is B.** (Mosby, *Patient Assessment.*) (B) is correct. (A), (C), and (D) are not indications for cervical spine immobilization.

112. The answer is D. (Mosby, *Patient Assessment.*) (A), (B), and (C) are correct. (D) is incorrect because a soft cervical collar is not an acceptable method of cervical spine immobilization.

113. The answer is B. (Mosby, *Patient Assessment.* Brady, *General Patient Assessment and Initial Management.*) Chest wall rise, normalization of heart rate, auscultation of lungs, respiratory rate, skin color, and pulse oximetry are appropriate techniques. (B) is incorrect because skin color changes can be an effective technique for evaluating the effectiveness of ventilation but not skin temperature.

114. The answer is C. (Mosby, *Patient Assessment.* Brady, *General Patient Assessment and Initial Management.*) (A), (B), (D), and checking for major bleeding are appropriate. (C) is incorrect because capillary refill is used primarily in children under age 6. There is controversy about its reliability in adults, particularly in some women and elderly patients.

115. The answer is D. (Mosby, *Patient Assessment.*) (A), (B), and (C) are correct. (D) is incorrect. The aorta is not considered a peripheral pulse and is not associated with a particular estimated systolic blood pressure.

116. The answer is A. (Mosby, *Patient Assessment.*) (A) is the correct definition. (B) is incorrect because VIPs (very important persons) are not a priority and should be treated according to the severity of illness. (C) and (D) are incorrect because stable patients by definition are stable and thus are not a priority.

117. The answer is A. (Mosby, *Patient Assessment.*) (B), (C) and (D) are clinical examples of priority patients. (A) is incorrect because responsive patients with stable vital signs and childbirth are not priority patients. A patient with difficulty breathing is a priority patient.

118. The answer is C. (Mosby, *Patient Assessment.*) (A), (B), and (D) are correct options used by various EMS medical controls for an EMT-I who is treating priority patients. (C) is incorrect because a high-speed ambulance ride should not be used for all priority patients because of the danger of inflicting further injuries from an ambulance accident.

119. The answer is D. (Mosby, *Patient Assessment.* Brady, *General Patient Assessment and Initial Management.*) (A), (B), (C), reassessing the patient's mental status, maintaining spinal immobilization, and obtaining baseline vital signs are all parts of the focused assessment. (D) is incorrect because beginning two large-bore intravenous lines is part of the initial treatment, not part of the assessment of a trauma patient.

120. The answer is D. (Mosby, *Patient Assessment.*) (A), (B), and (C) are correct. (D) is incorrect because the normal range for an adult is 90-140 mm Hg systolic and 60-90 mm Hg diastolic.

121. The answer is D. (Brady, *General Patient Assessment and Initial Management.*) Establishing an airway is the first priority in this trauma patient, using cervical spine precautions. (A), (B), and (C) are all very important parts of the treatment of a trauma patient, but establishing the airway is the first priority.

122. The answer is A. (Mosby, *Patient Assessment.*) (B), (C), and (D) are correct. (A) is incorrect because the normal respiratory rate in a newborn is 40 breaths per minute.

123. The answer is C. (Mosby, *Patient Assessment.*) (A), (B), and (D) are correct. In an adult, the normal pulse rate is 60–100 beats per minute. (C) is incorrect because the normal pulse rate in an older child (8 to 12 years) is 55–110 beats per minute.

124. The answer is C. (Mosby, *Patient Assessment.*) (A), (B), and (D) are correct. (C) is incorrect because the administration of intravenous narcan is not part of a focused examination of this patient.

125. Answers. (Mosby, *Patient Assessment.*)
O = onset
P = provocation
Q = quality
R = radiation
S = severity
T = time

126. The answer is C. (Mosby, *Patient Assessment.*) (A), (B), and (D) make up the detailed assessment. (C) is incorrect because this is not considered part of the detailed assessment.

127. The answer is D. (Mosby, *Patient Assessment.*) (D) is correct because a detailed assessment may reveal a cause of the fall, such as syncope, as well as other potentially critical injuries. (A) is incorrect because a detailed assessment is not indicated for a simple fingertip laceration. (B) and (C) are incorrect because these patients could benefit from a detailed assessment performed during transport to the hospital. This should not be done on the scene.

128. The answer is D. (Mosby, *Patient Assessment.*) (A), (B), and (C) are correct. (D) is incorrect because the range of eye opening is 4 to 1.

129. The answer is C. (Mosby, *Patient Assessment.*) (A), (B), and (D) are all parts of an ongoing assessment. (C) is incorrect because while one may choose to perform all these tasks, they are not considered parts of an ongoing assessment.

130. The answer is D. (Mosby, *Patient Assessment.*) (D) is correct. (A), (B), and (C) are all incorrect.

131. The answer is C. (Mosby, *Patient Assessment.*) (A), (B), and (D) are correct. In many emergency medical systems the EMT-I determines the facility on the basis of written protocols or medical control authorization. (C) is incorrect because while a patient's medical records are very important for the proper care of the patient, they are not required in determining the facility.

132. The answer is A. (Mosby, *Patient Assessment.*) (B), (C), (D), the number of patients transported, the care being rendered, and the results of the care rendered are all parts of the essential information which has to be communicated. (A) is incorrect because knowing the next of kin is helpful but not as important as the previously stated information.

133. The answer is B. (Mosby, *Patient Assessment.*) (A), (C), and (D) are all correct reasons for providing accurate documentation. (B) is incorrect because it has nothing to do with accurate documentation.

AIRWAY
MANAGEMENT

In this chapter, you will review:

- anatomy of the adult airway

- airway assessment

- airway opening and maintenance maneuvers

AIRWAY MANAGEMENT

Directions: Each item below contains four suggested responses. Select the **one best** response to each item.

134. In the adult airway label the following: nasopharynx, oropharynx, laryngopharynx, epiglottis, larynx, trachea, true vocal cord, vestibular fold, thyroid cartilage, and the cricoid cartilage.

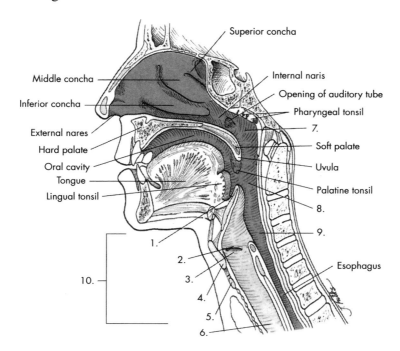

Adapted from Mosby: *EMT-Intermediate Textbook*, Mosby-Lifeline, 1997, with permission.

135. All of the following are regions of the pharynx EXCEPT

   (A) nasopharynx
   (B) pharyngeal pharynx
   (C) oropharynx
   (D) laryngopharynx

136. Which of the following statements describes the main difference between the true and false vocal cords?

   (A) The true vocal cords control the act of speaking, while the false cords control the act of singing
   (B) The true vocal cords are located above the false cords
   (C) The true vocal cords control the passage of air through the pharynx and the production of sound
   (D) The true vocal cords are located in the nasopharynx, and the false vocal cords are located in the oropharynx

137. Identify and label the tongue, esophagus, true vocal cord, vestibular fold (false vocal cord), epiglottis, cricoid cartilage, trachea, and thyroid cartilage.

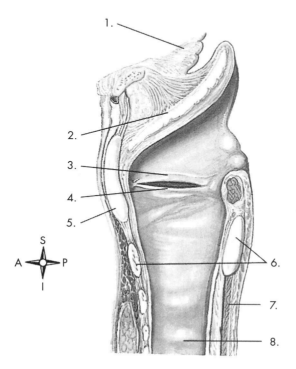

Adapted from Shade, Rothenberg, Wertz, and Jones: *Mosby's EMT-Intermediate Textbook*, Mosby-Lifeline, 1997, with permission.

138. On the blank lines, label the correct anatomic areas for the nasopharynx, oropharynx, and laryngopharynx.

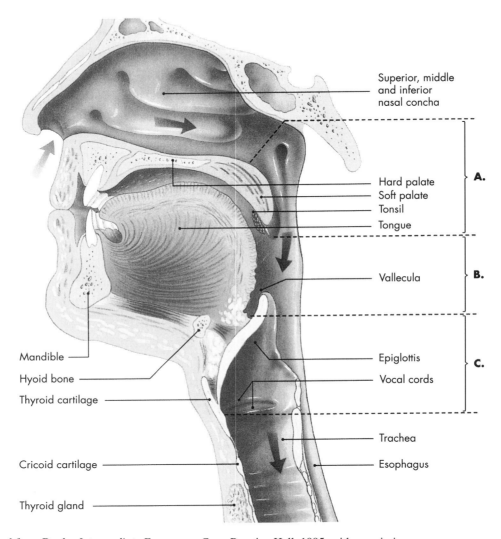

Adapted from Brady: *Intermediate Emergency Care*, Prentice-Hall, 1995, with permission.

139. An EMT-I arrives at the scene of a motor vehicle accident and finds a 30-year-old male trapped in the driver's seat and unconscious. Which of the following is the correct way to assess the patient's airway?

(A) Auscultate both lungs anteriorly and posteriorly
(B) Look at the skin surface of the anterior neck, which covers the airway, for signs of trauma
(C) Check the pulse and blood pressure as indicators
(D) Look, listen, and feel for airway movement and sounds

140. After establishing an airway for a 30-year-old motor vehicle accident patient, an EMT-I immediately begins to assess the adequacy of the patient's ventilation. All of the following are used to assure the adequacy of the patient's ventilation EXCEPT

(A) assessment of the level of consciousness and leg edema
(B) airway patency and neck appearance
(C) skin color, auscultation of lung sounds, pulse rate
(D) chest silence and lung compliance to bagging with bag-valve-mask device

141. In using pulse oximetry to assess the level of oxygenation, the following ranges of oxygen saturation (Sa_{O_2}) are correct EXCEPT

(A) Sa_{O_2} less than 85% represents moderate hypoxemia
(B) Sa_{O_2} 95–99% is ideal
(C) Sa_{O_2} 91–94% shows mild hypoxemia
(D) Sa_{O_2} 85–90% represents moderate hypoxemia

142. In using pulse oximetry, an EMT-I must realize that many circumstances produce false readings. All of the following produce false readings EXCEPT

(A) carbon monoxide
(B) fingernail polish
(C) hypotension
(D) high blood pressure

143. All of the following list causes of upper airway obstruction and maneuvers to attempt to relieve it EXCEPT

(A) tongue and epiglottis obstruction may be relieved by head tilt/chin lift, jaw thrust maneuver, or jaw lift maneuver alone

(B) foreign body and tooth obstruction may be relieved by direct visualization and removal or the Heimlich maneuver

(C) vomitus and blood obstruction may be relieved by head tilt/chin lift, jaw thrust maneuver, or jaw lift maneuver alone

(D) airway swelling from an allergic reaction or smoke inhalation may be relieved by head tilt/chin lift, jaw thrust maneuver, or jaw lift maneuver. However, EMT-Paramedics (EMT-Ps) or Emergency Department physicians may be needed to provide an airway below the upper airway, such as needle cricothyrotomy, or a tracheotomy

144. All of the following are correct steps in performing the head tilt/chin lift maneuver to open the airway EXCEPT

(A) use body substance isolation precautions

(B) place uppermost hand on patient's forehead with downward pressure by the palm to tilt patient's head back

(C) grasp patient's chin with other hand's thumb on front of jaw and index finger under patient's jaw

(D) lift jaw inferiorly to open airway

145. All of the following are correct steps in performing the jaw thrust maneuver to open the airway EXCEPT

(A) use body substance isolation precautions

(B) position oneself at top of patient's head with elbows resting on each side of the floor

(C) place fingertips on each side of patient's forehead

(D) firmly push jaw forward while tilting head back and retracting patient's lower lip with both thumbs

146. All of the following are correct steps in performing the jaw lift maneuver to open the airway EXCEPT

(A) use body substance isolation precautions

(B) use one hand to grasp the mandible by placing the thumb deep into the mouth, pressing down on the tongue, and placing the index finger under the mandible

(C) lift the jaw anteriorly to open the airway

(D) jaw lift should be the airway's opening maneuver of choice in a trauma patient

147. You are returning from the gas station, and two women flag you down to look at a 60-year-old man who passed out in the bank. As you arrive on the main floor of the bank, you find the patient unresponsive with snoring respirations and a strong pulse. Because the witnesses stated that the patient passed out and hit his head on the floor, you carefully proceed to open the airway with a chin lift maneuver, with the head kept in a neutral position. As you consider a way to maintain the open airway, the use of an oropharyngeal airway is considered. All of the following are true concerning the use of an oropharyngeal airway (OPA) EXCEPT

(A) the main indication is to maintain an open airway in an unresponsive, breathing patient without a gag reflex

(B) another indication is to maintain an open airway in a patient who is being ventilated with a bag-valve-mask or another pressure device

(C) the main contraindication to its use is a patient with a gag reflex because an OPA can trigger cardiac arrhythmias

(D) another contraindication is a patient with severe maxillofacial injuries

148. All of the following are parts of the process of inserting an OPA EXCEPT

(A) a properly sized OPA will go from the mouth to the angle of the patient's jaw

(B) after opening the airway, grasp the patient's tongue and jaw to lift them anteriorly; then insert the OPA with the tip pointing to the roof of the mouth

(C) at the middle of the tongue, turn the OPA 180° until it rests over the tongue

(D) check for proper position of the OPA by listening for clear breath sounds and chest rise

149. All of the following are true concerning the use of a nasopharyngeal airway EXCEPT

(A) it is indicated to relieve soft tissue upper airway obstruction when an OPA is contraindicated

(B) a contraindication to its use is any evidence of nasal obstruction or a patient with a history of nose-bleeds

(C) another contraindication is suspicion of an occipital skull fracture (back of the skull)

(D) it may be used in a patient with a positive gag reflex

150. All of the following are true statements concerning the use of the esophageal obturator airway (EOA) EXCEPT

    (A) while an endotracheal tube is used in an unconscious patient without a gag reflex, an EOA can be used in a conscious patient with a positive gag reflex

    (B) an EOA is an alternative to the endotracheal tube for personnel who are not trained, permitted, or able to use an endotracheal tube

    (C) the proximal end of an EOA is open, and the distal end is closed

    (D) an EOA may be used in trauma victims with possible spinal injuries because there is no need to hyperextend or flex the neck with insertion

151. In proceeding to insert an EOA, which of the following is a true statement?

    (A) Contraindications to using an EOA include persons under age 16 and persons who may have ingested caustic poisons

    (B) After inserting an EOA into the esophagus, connect the face mask

    (C) When inserting an EOA, if there is any resistance, rotate the tube and apply more pressure

    (D) After successfully inserting an EOA, if there are breath sounds and chest rise, inflate the distal cuff with 10–15 mL of air

152. In deciding whether to use an EOA or an esophageal gastric tube airway (EGTA) to secure a patient's airway, all of the following points are true EXCEPT

    (A) the technique for inserting an EGTA is the same as that for an EOA

    (B) the indications and contraindications for its use are the same as those for an EOA

    (C) the primary difference between the two tubes is that an EGTA is inserted into the stomach instead of the esophagus

    (D) the transparent face mask has two parts: one to allow attachment to the esophageal tube and the other to serve as a ventilation port

153. You have been trained and authorized to use a pharyngotracheal lumen airway (PTL). As you consider using it, which of the following is a true statement concerning the PTL?

    (A) It is inserted, like an endotracheal tube, with a laryngoscope blade

    (B) Like an EOA and an EGTA, it must be inserted only into the esophagus

    (C) A PTL prevents the patient from aspirating foreign materials (blood or vomit) from the upper airway when the longer tube is in the esophagus

    (D) After insertion, one connects a ventilatory device to the green tube and delivers a breath. If the chest rises, the longer tube is in the esophagus and ventilations should be continued through the green tube

154. You are dispatched to a nursing home to see a 75-year-old patient in cardiac arrest. As you arrive at the bedside, you find the patient apneic and pulseless. After a quick look with your automatic external defibrillator (AED), you note that the rhythm is asystole. As your partner begins cardiopulmonary resuscitation (CPR), you consider the best means of providing airway protection and ventilation. Which of the following is the BEST method?

(A) Pharyngotracheal airway
(B) Bag-valve-mask with oxygen
(C) Esophageal obturator airway
(D) Endotracheal tube intubation

155. All of the following statements are true concerning the technique of suctioning the upper airway EXCEPT

(A) suctioning is indicated to clear the upper airway of vomitus, blood, fluids, and secretions
(B) each suctioning attempt should be restricted to 15 seconds or less
(C) the whistle-tip catheter is designed to remove larger particles and larger volumes of secretions than is the tonsil-tip catheter
(D) the patient should be hyperventilated with 100% oxygen before and after suctioning

156. You are dispatched to a 90-year-old weak female with recurrent vomiting. As you begin to assess the patient, you find her weak and lethargic with gurgling respirations. After noting stable vital signs, you begin to suction the secretions but are unable to do so because of their thickness. Your next step should be to

(A) take a quick look with an AED
(B) turn the patient on her side and perform back blows
(C) insert an OPA and try to suction through it
(D) remove the catheter and use the thick-walled, wide-bore suction tubing itself

157. Which of the following would be an indication for providing assisted ventilation in a patient with ventilatory failure?

(A) Blood pressure 100/60 and pulse of 120 per minute
(B) Temperature of 103° with lethargy
(C) Respiratory rate less than 10 or more than 30 breaths per minute
(D) A trauma patient with a respiratory rate of 16 per minute

158. All of the following are causes of ventilatory failure EXCEPT

(A) spinal injury, head injury, and flail chest
(B) pneumothorax, fractured ribs, and drug overdose
(C) diabetes and hypertension
(D) asthma and chronic obstructive pulmonary disease (COPD)

159. You arrive at the home of a 68-year-old female three-pack-a-day smoker with COPD who is demonstrating respiratory failure and breathing eight times a minute. As you assist the patient's ventilations, you think about certain characteristics of the pocket mask. All of the following statements are true EXCEPT

(A) mouth-to-mask breathing supplemented with oxygen attached at a flow rate of 10 liters per minute will deliver an oxygen concentration of 50%

(B) pocket masks have one-way valves that prevent a prehospital provider from coming in contact with the patient's expired air

(C) the pocket mask is applied by placing the wide end over the bridge of the nose and the narrow end over the chin

(D) mouth-to-mask breathing has been found to be more effective than is bag-valve-mask breathing

160. You are dispatched to the scene of a "difficulty breathing" patient. As you arrive, you find a 78-year-old male patient who is breathing at a rate of six times per minute. The family states that he has a chronic lung disease (emphysema) and has had increasing difficulty breathing for the past 2 days. In deciding to help the patient breathe, you select a bag-valve-mask device. All of the following statements are true concerning the use of a bag-valve-mask device EXCEPT

(A) to adequately ventilate the patient, you must deliver 800 to 1200 mL of air per breath

(B) in the prehospital community this is accepted as always being a very easy device to use

(C) one of the most difficult aspects of using this device is keeping a tight seal to the face while maintaining an open airway

(D) with supplemental oxygen attached at 15 liters per minute, a bag-valve-mask can deliver 40–60% oxygen

161. All of the following are true statements about the use of a demand valve resuscitator EXCEPT

(A) it will deliver 100% oxygen at its highest flow rate of 40 liters per minute

(B) it may not be used in spontaneously breathing patients

(C) a contraindication to its use is a patient less than 16 years of age

(D) because of the sudden high pressures from this device, it should be used with extreme caution in intubated patients and chest trauma patients

162. In using a demand valve device, high-pressured oxygen is delivered to the patient by which of the following means?

(A) Touching the mouth with the demand valve triggers oxygen release

(B) Squeezing the bag-valve-mask device triggers oxygen release

(C) Dialing the correct oxygen concentration on the demand valve triggers oxygen release

(D) Pushing the button on the device triggers oxygen release

163. All of the following are mechanisms of hypoxia EXCEPT

(A) insufficient oxygen in inspired air as a result of epiglottitis, croup, or foreign body airway obstruction

(B) failure of the ventilatory mechanism as a result of fractured ribs, pneumothorax, or kyphoscoliosis

(C) failure of the circulation mechanism as a result of congestive heart failure, shock, or hemorrhage

(D) lower airway compromise caused by chronic bronchitis, emphysema, asthma, or tumor

164. You arrive at the scene of a fire and are asked to assess a 70-year-old male patient with known chronic bronchitis. The patient states that he walked quickly down four flights of stairs and feels a little short of breath. Your assessment reveals a 70-year-old male breathing 22 times a minute, in no acute distress, with clear lung sounds, and not using any accessory muscles. This patient should be given supplemental oxygen by which of the following techniques?

(A) Endotracheal intubation with a demand valve device delivering 100% oxygen

(B) A nasal cannula delivering 24–44% oxygen at 1–3 liters per minute

(C) A bag-valve-mask with a reservoir to deliver 85–100% oxygen

(D) A demand valve mask device to deliver 100% oxygen at 40 liters per minute

165. You are dispatched to a 54-year-old man with severe chest pain. As you arrive at the patient's side, he admits to having had severe substernal chest pain for 2 hours, with radiation to his arms bilaterally. He also admits to sweating, palpitations, shortness of breath, and nausea. He has high blood pressure and has smoked two packs per day for 32 years. As your partner starts to assess the patient, you begin to consider administering oxygen to the patient. Which is the correct way to administer oxygen to this patient?

(A) A non-rebreather mask with nasal O_2 attached at 10–15 liters per minute, which can deliver 80–100% oxygen concentration

(B) A Venturi mask set at 28% oxygen concentration

(C) A nasal cannula at 6 liters per minute delivering 44% oxygen concentration

(D) A simple face mask at 8–12 liters per minute delivering 40–60% oxygen concentration

166. Venturi masks are designed to allow dial selection of oxygen concentration to be delivered to the patient. All of the following are possible oxygen concentrations which may be selected EXCEPT

(A) 24%

(B) 28%

(C) 40%

(D) 60%

167. All of the following are indications for the use of endotracheal intubation EXCEPT

(A) the EMT-I is unable to ventilate an unresponsive patient with conventional means

(B) the patient cannot protect the airway (e.g., coma or cardiac or respiratory arrest)

(C) an unresponsive patient without a gag reflex

(D) an asthmatic patient in mild respiratory distress who has run out of bronchodilator inhaler medication

168. In the early stages of preparing to perform endotracheal intubation, which of the following is the correct sequence?

(A) Body isolation precautions, airway-opening maneuver, hyperventilate with 100% oxygen, partner or First Responder ventilates the patient

(B) Assemble and check the equipment, hyperventilate with 100% oxygen, open the airway

(C) Airway-opening maneuvers, body isolation precautions, assemble and check the equipment, hyperventilate with 100% oxygen

(D) Hyperventilate with 100% oxygen, assemble and check the equipment, airway-opening maneuvers

169. All of the following are parts of the equipment used to perform endotracheal intubation EXCEPT

(A) laryngoscope with accessories
(B) 10-mL syringe, stylet, endotracheal tubes
(C) nasal cannula, Venturi mask
(D) bite block, suction device, Magill forceps

170. After using body isolation precautions, opening the airway, and then hyperventilating the patient with 100% oxygen while your partner or the First Responder ventilates the patient, you continue to perform endotracheal intubation in which of the following sequences?

(A) Manipulate the laryngoscope blade into position, align the head and neck in the correct position, check the endotracheal tube placement
(B) Place the endotracheal tube into the glottic opening and then manipulate the laryngoscope blade into the proper position
(C) Align the head and neck in the correct position, manipulate the laryngoscope blade into the proper position, with the right hand insert the endotracheal tube into the glottic opening, inflate the distal cuff with 5–10 mL of air
(D) Align the head and neck in the correct position, check the endotracheal tube placement, manipulate the laryngoscope blade into the proper position

171. All of the following are techniques for verifying correct placement of an endotracheal tube EXCEPT

(A) listen for bilateral lung sounds and the absence of breath sounds over the epigastrium
(B) check for condensation in the proximal end of the tube during each exhalation
(C) revisualize the endotracheal tube going past the vocal cords
(D) attach pulse oximetry to the end of the patient's finger

AIRWAY MANAGEMENT

ANSWERS

134. Answers.

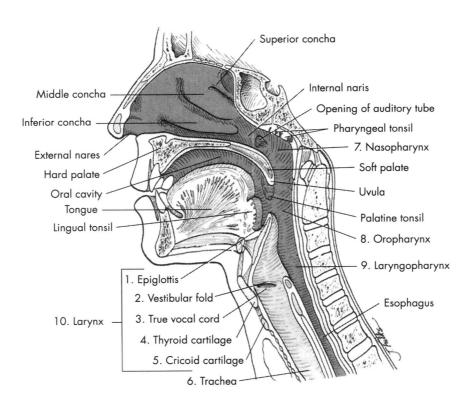

Adapted from Mosby: *EMT-Intermediate Textbook*, Mosby-Lifeline, 1997, with permission.

135. **The answer is B.** (Mosby, *Airway Management.*) (A), (C), and (D) are regions of the pharynx. (B) is not.

136. **The answer is C.** (Brady, *Airway Management and Ventilation.*) The true vocal cords are located below the false vocal cords. Both are located in the laryngopharynx.

137. Answers.

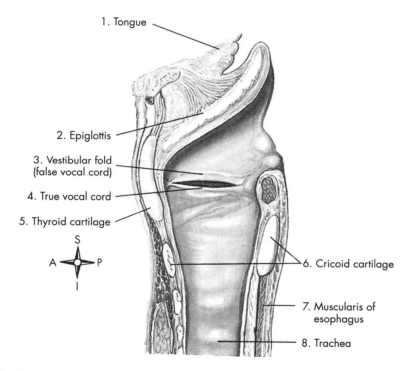

1. Tongue
2. Epiglottis
3. Vestibular fold (false vocal cord)
4. True vocal cord
5. Thyroid cartilage
6. Cricoid cartilage
7. Muscularis of esophagus
8. Trachea

Adapted from Shade, Rothenberg, Wertz, and Jones: Mosby's *EMT-Intermediate Textbook*, Mosby-Lifeline, 1997, with permission.

138. Answers.

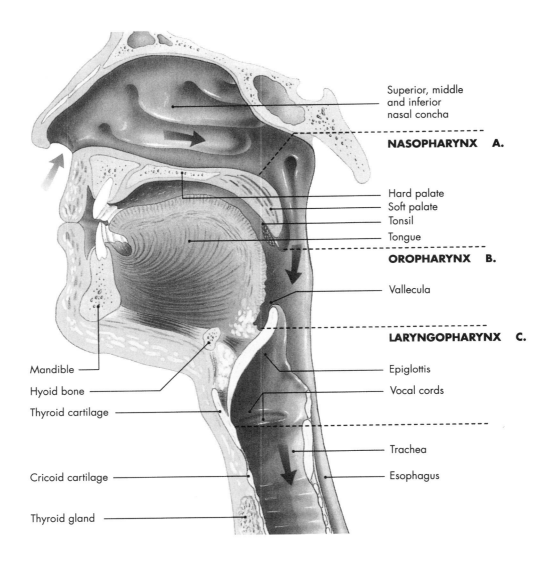

Adapted from Brady, *Intermediate Emergency Care*, Prentice-Hall, 1995, with permission.

139. The answer is D. (Mosby, *Airway Management.*) (A) is incorrect because this is part of the process of evaluating a patient's ventilation. (B) is incorrect because the neck can provide clues to ventilation problems such as tracheal deviation, distended neck veins, and tracheal tugging. (C) is incorrect because the pulse and blood pressure are used to assess the circulation, not the airway.

140. The answer is A. (Mosby, *Airway Management.*) (B), (C), and (D) are all methods of assessing the adequacy of ventilation. (A) is incorrect because the level of consciousness may vary between full alertness and unconsciousness in a patient with ventilatory problems. Leg edema is not related to ventilation.

141. The answer is A. (Mosby, *Airway Management.*) (B), (C), and (D) are correct. (A) is incorrect because an Sa_{O_2} less than 85% represents severe hypoxemia.

142. The answer is D. (Mosby, *Airway Management.*) (A), (B), (C), patient movement, hypothermia, jaundice, the use of vasoactive drugs, and excessive ambient light can all produce false readings of oxygen saturation (Sa_{O_2}). High blood pressure does not affect oxygen saturation.

143. The answer is C. (Mosby, *Airway Management.*) (A), (B), and (D) list examples of upper airway obstruction and correct methods to relieve it. (C) is incorrect because usually both vomitus and blood require suctioning in addition to airway-opening maneuvers.

144. The answer is D. (Mosby, *Airway Management.*) (A), (B), and (C) are correct. (D) is incorrect because in the last step one lifts the jaw anteriorly to open the airway.

145. The answer is C. (Mosby, *Airway Management.*) (A), (B), and (D) are correct steps. (C) is incorrect because one should place the fingertips on each side of the patient's lower jaw.

146. The answer is D. (Mosby, *Airway Management.*) (A), (B), and (C) are correct. (D) is incorrect because the jaw lift maneuver should never be used in a trauma patient. For a trauma patient with a suspected spine injury, one should use the chin lift or jaw thrust maneuver without head tilt.

147. The answer is C. (Mosby, *Airway Management.*) (A), (B), and (D) are correct. The OPA is also indicated for use as a bite block to prevent patients from biting an endotracheal tube and thus occluding it. (C) is incorrect because while it is contraindicated to use an OPA in a patient with a gag reflex, the reason for this is that the OPA may cause vomiting or laryngospasm. It does not cause cardiac arrhythmias.

148. The answer is C. (Brady, *Airway Management and Ventilation.*) (A), (B), and (D) are parts of the process. (C) is incorrect because one rotates the OPA 180° at the level of the uvula, not at the middle of the tongue.

149. The answer is C. (Brady, *Airway Management and Ventilation.*) (A), (B) and (D) are correct. (C) is incorrect because a suspicion of a basilar skull fracture is a contraindication to the use of a nasopharyngeal airway. With the presence of a basilar skull fracture, one may pass the nasopharyngeal airway into the brain. With an occipital skull fracture, the EMT-I may use the nasopharyngeal airway, without fear of passing it into the brain.

150. The answer is A. (Brady, *Airway Management and Ventilation.*) (B), (C), and (D) are correct. (A) is incorrect because an EOA can be used only in an unconscious patient, without a gag reflex. If a patient regains consciousness with a positive gag reflex, the EOA must be removed.

151. The answer is A. (Brady, *Airway Management and Ventilation.*) (B) is incorrect because before inserting an EOA, one connects the tube to the face mask. (C) is incorrect because while inserting an EOA, if one encounters any resistance, one should withdraw the tube and try again. (D) is incorrect because after a successful insertion, the distal cuff is inflated with 30–35 mL of air.

152. The answer is C. (Brady, *Airway Management and Ventilation.*) (C) is incorrect because the primary difference between the two tubes is that an EGTA is open throughout its length to allow the passage of a gastric tube to decompress the stomach.

153. The answer is D. (Brady, *Airway Management and Ventilation.*) (A) is incorrect because a PTL is inserted blindly and does not require visualization of the upper airway. (B) is incorrect because a PTL may be inserted into the esophagus or the trachea. (C) is incorrect because when the longer tube is in the esophagus, the device does not keep the patient from aspirating materials from the upper airway.

154. The answer is D. (Mosby, *Airway Management.*) (A), (B) and (C) are all very good alternatives for managing the airway and ventilating the patient. However, (D) is the best option.

155. The answer is C. (Mosby, *Airway Management.*) (A), (B) and (D) are correct. (C) is incorrect because the tonsil-tip catheter is designed to remove larger particles and larger volumes of secretions than is the smaller whistle-tip catheter.

156. The answer is D. (Mosby, *Airway Management.*) (A) is incorrect because the patient is not in cardiac arrest, and therefore there is no indication for the use of an AED. (B) is incorrect because turning the patient on her side and using the fingers to clear the airway sometimes is an alternative to suctioning the airway. (C) is incorrect because one never inserts an OPA in a responsive patient with a positive gag reflex.

157. The answer is C. (Mosby, *Airway Management.*) A patient with ventilatory failure with a respiratory rate less than 10 or more than 30 breaths per minute requires assisted ventilations. This may be provided by mouth-to-mouth/nose breathing, mouth-to-mask breathing, a bag-valve-mask device, a demand-valve resuscitator, or an automatic ventilator.

158. The answer is C. (Mosby, *Airway Management.*) (A), (B), (D), muscular paralysis, and poliomyelitis are all causes of ventilatory failure. Diabetes and hypertension are not.

159. The answer is C. (Mosby, *Airway Management.*) (C) is incorrect because the correct way to apply a pocket mask is to place the narrow end over the bridge of the nose and the wide end in the groove between the lower lip and the chin.

160. The answer is B. (Mosby, *Airway Management.*) (A), (C) and (D) are correct. (B) is incorrect because despite its increased use in the prehospital setting, a bag-valve-mask device is well known for being difficult to use. The main problems are maintaining a tight seal and an open airway and compressing the bag sufficiently to ventilate the patient. Ventilation with a bag-valve-mask may be more effectively performed by two EMT-Intermediates (EMT-Is).

161. **The answer is B.** (Brady, *Airway Management and Ventilation.*) (A), (C), and (D) are correct. (B) is incorrect because a demand valve device contains an inspiratory release valve which permits a spontaneously breathing patient to use it.

162. **The answer is D.** (Mosby, *Airway Management.*) When using body substance isolation precautions, one applies the correct size face mask, using both hands to make a tight seal, while hyperextending the neck (except in trauma patients). The demand valve device delivers high-pressured oxygen when one pushes the button on the top of the device.

163. **The answer is A.** (Mosby, *Airway Management.*) (B), (C), and (D) are correct. (A) is incorrect because insufficient oxygen in inspired air is due to smoke, high altitude, or toxic gases. Upper airway compromise is due to epiglottitis, croup, foreign body obstruction and vocal cord edema. Cellular deficiency is due to cyanide poisoning and toxic shock syndrome.

164. **The answer is B.** (Brady, *Airway Management and Ventilation.* Mosby, *Airway Management.*) Since this patient probably is demonstrating mild to moderate hypoxia and is breathing well on his own, (B) is the correct answer. (A), (C), and (D) are incorrect because these procedures are used primarily in patients demonstrating inadequate ventilations and requiring assisted ventilation. Also, in a stable patient with chronic bronchitis, one should try to avoid ventilatory devices which deliver high concentration oxygen, which could suppress this patient's hypoxic drive to breathe and cause retention of carbon dioxide (CO_2).

165. **The answer is A.** (Brady, *Airway Management and Ventilation.*) (A) is correct because for any patient with possible severe hypoxia, such as an acute myocardial infarction, shock, respiratory insufficiency, trauma, or carbon monoxide poisoning, you must try to administer 80–100% oxygen concentration. (B), (C), and (D) are all incorrect because you must try to administer 80–100% oxygen concentration. However, sometimes patients adamantly refuse all face masks yet will accept a nasal cannula, which is better than the room air oxygen concentration of 21%.

166. **The answer is D.** (Brady, *Airway Management and Ventilation.*) Venturi masks can be dial selected to deliver oxygen concentrations of 24%, 28%, 35%, and 40%. They cannot deliver an oxygen concentration of 60%.

167. **The answer is D.** (Mosby, *Airway Management.*) (A), (B), (C), the need for prolonged ventilation, patients experiencing or likely to experience upper airway compromise, decreased tidal volume caused by slow respirations, and airway obstruction resulting from foreign bodies, trauma, or anaphylaxis are all indications for endotracheal intubation. (D) is incorrect because asthmatic patients in mild respiratory distress should be treated with aerosol bronchodilator inhaler medications and then should be considered for oral or intravenous steroids as the first line of treatment. Endotracheal intubation may be indicated in asthmatic patients who have the indications outlined above for its use.

168. The answer is A. (Mosby, *Airway Management.*) (A) is the correct sequence. (B), (C), and (D) are all incorrect.

169. The answer is C. (Brady, *Airway Management and Ventilation.*) (A), (B), (D), face and eye protection, a bag-valve device, and a tape- or tube-holding device are all parts of the equipment used for endotracheal intubation. (C) lists two oxygen-delivering devices that are not used as endotracheal intubation equipment.

170. The answer is C. (Brady, *Airway Management and Ventilation.*) (C) is the correct sequence. (A), (B), and (D) are incorrect.

171. The answer is D. (Mosby, *Airway Management.*) (A), (B), (C), end-tidal carbon dioxide disposable detectors, and electronic monitors are all used to verify correct endotracheal tube placement. (D) is incorrect because the oxygen saturation detected by pulse oximetry cannot be used to verify endotracheal tube placement.

ASSESSMENT
AND MANAGEMENT
OF SHOCK

In this chapter, you will review:

- aerobic and anaerobic metabolism
- role of fluid intake
- five types of shock

ASSESSMENT AND MANAGEMENT OF SHOCK

Directions: Each item below contains four suggested responses. Select the **one best** response to each item.

172. All of the following are true statements concerning the differences between aerobic and anaerobic cellular metabolism EXCEPT

   (A) anaerobic metabolism occurs in poor perfusion states with hypoxia
   (B) aerobic metabolism occurs with the combination of oxygen and glucose
   (C) aerobic metabolism results in a buildup of pyruvic acid which degrades to lactic acid
   (D) aerobic metabolism results in the production of carbon dioxide

173. Which of the following is the best definition of perfusion?

   (A) The process of intravenous fluid being delivered to the body
   (B) The process by which oxygenated blood is delivered to the body's tissues and wastes are removed
   (C) The process by which there is a normal buildup of lactic acid
   (D) The process by which a dialysis machine removes waste products and returns red blood cells to the body

174. All of the following are elements of the Fick principle concerning oxygen transport EXCEPT

(A) an adequate concentration of inspired oxygen
(B) diffusion of oxygen across the alveolar-capillary membrane
(C) an adequate number of white blood cells to carry oxygen and adequate perfusion
(D) off-loading of oxygen at the tissue level

175. Which of the following is the best definition of the cardiovascular system?

(A) A system of arteries, capillaries, and veins
(B) A system consisting of the heart, brain, and kidneys
(C) A system in which the heart moves blood throughout the body in a closed system of blood vessels
(D) A system in which the heart moves blood throughout the body in an open delivery system of oxygen

176. All of the following affect the heart's function as the lead organ in the body's cardiovascular system EXCEPT

(A) stroke volume
(B) preload
(C) afterload
(D) skin pallor

177. All of the following are blood vessels in the cardiovascular system EXCEPT

(A) bronchi and bronchioles
(B) arteries and arterioles
(C) veins and venules
(D) aorta and inferior and superior venae cavae

178. All of the following statements are true concerning the role of water in the body EXCEPT

(A) next to fat and the subcutaneous tissue, it is the second most abundant substance in the body
(B) it plays a very important role in maintaining homeostasis in the body
(C) it functions as a solvent for various solutions in the body, such as electrolytes
(D) in the average adult, body water content is about 50–60 percent of total body weight

179. The fluid compartments of the body consist of all of the following EXCEPT

(A) intracellular fluid accounts for 40–45 percent of total body weight and 75 percent of all body fluid
(B) extracellular fluid accounts for 40–45 percent of total body weight and 75 percent of all body fluid
(C) intravascular fluid accounts for 4.5 percent of total body weight
(D) interstitial fluid accounts for 10.5 percent of total body weight

180. All of the following are significant cations in the body EXCEPT

(A) sodium (Na^+)
(B) potassium (K^+)
(C) calcium (Ca^{2+})
(D) cadmium (Cd^{2+})

181. All of the following are significant anions in the body EXCEPT

(A) chloride (Cl^-)
(B) bicarbonate (HCO_3^-)
(C) sulfate (SO_4^-)
(D) phosphate (HPO_4^-)

182. Which of the following is a true statement about the semipermeable nature of the cell membrane?

(A) The first half of the membrane allows water and nutrients through, while the back half is nonpermeable
(B) The cell membrane allows water and nutrients to penetrate but not leave
(C) The cell membrane allows nutrients but not water to penetrate
(D) The cell membrane allows some substances but not others to enter and leave the cell

183. Match the following definitions with the correct concepts:

(A) Diffusion _____
(B) Facilitated diffusion _____
(C) Osmosis _____
(D) Osmotic pressure _____
(E) Active transport _____

1. Movement of a solute across a membrane from a low concentration to a high concentration
2. Movement of particles from an area of high concentration to an area of low concentration
3. A specialized transport protein binds to a molecule of another substance and moves across a cell membrane
4. The movement of water across a semipermeable membrane
5. A hypotonic solution has less and a hypertonic solution has more than normal body fluids

184. All of the following are examples of fluids with a certain tonicity EXCEPT

(A) 0.9% normal saline is isotonic
(B) lactated Ringer's solution is isotonic
(C) dextrose in water (D_5W) is hypotonic
(D) 5% saline is isotonic

185. Match the following blood products with the correct functions:

(A) Plasma _____
(B) Erythrocytes _____
(C) Leukocytes _____
(D) Platelets _____
(E) Hemoglobin _____
(F) Hematocrit _____

   1. Most numerous blood cells which carry oxygen
   2. Iron-based protein which binds oxygen to red blood cells
   3. The fluid or water portion of blood
   4. Destroy bacteria
   5. Volume of red blood cells in whole blood
   6. Suspended in plasma and important in blood clotting

186. All of the following are correct statements about antigens EXCEPT

(A) an antigen is a protein found on the membrane of a red blood cell which causes the production of antibodies
(B) type A blood has type A surface antigens
(C) type B blood has type B surface antigens
(D) type O blood has type O surface antigens

187. All of the following are true statements about antibodies EXCEPT

(A) an antibody is a protein in the body which develops in response to an antigen
(B) type A blood has anti-B antibodies and will clump in type B blood
(C) type AB blood has anti-A and anti-B antibodies
(D) type O blood has anti-A and anti-B antibodies and patients with type O blood can receive only type O blood

188. All of the following are true statements concerning the Rh factor EXCEPT

(A) 85 percent of persons in the United States are Rh-negative
(B) a patient must receive blood from a donor with the same Rh factor
(C) all patients are either Rh-positive or Rh-negative
(D) Rh factor is an antigen on the red blood cell membrane

189. The pH of the human body is a balance between the amount of acid produced and the amount eliminated. All of the following affect the pH of the body EXCEPT

(A) an acid increases the hydrogen ion concentration of water and has a pH less than 7.0

(B) a base decreases the hydrogen ion concentration of water and has a pH greater than 7.0

(C) the pH of the human body is usually 7.25–7.35

(D) the three principal mechanisms for maintaining the body's pH are buffer systems, the lungs, and the kidneys

190. Buffer systems are available to help maintain acid-base balance throughout the body. All of the following are correct statements about the body's buffer systems EXCEPT

(A) these buffer systems are slow-acting and often require several days to produce an effect

(B) the body's major buffer system is the bicarbonate–carbonic acid buffer system

(C) normally there are 20 parts bicarbonate to 1 part carbonic acid

(D) when a strong acid enters the body, bicarbonate combines with it to produce a weak acid—carbonic acid—per the following formula:

$$H^+ + HCO_3^- \longleftrightarrow H_2CO_3$$
$$\longleftrightarrow H_2O + CO_2$$

191. All of the following are true statements concerning the role of the respiratory system in maintaining acid-base balance in the body EXCEPT

(A) it acts primarily by regulating the carbon dioxide concentration in the body

(B) increased ventilation decreases carbon dioxide and carbonic acid in the blood, which raises blood pH

(C) decreased ventilation increases carbon dioxide and carbonic acid in the blood, which decreases blood pH

(D) patients who have metabolic acidosis (e.g., diabetic ketoacidosis) compensate by retaining carbon dioxide

192. All of the following are correct statements concerning the role of the kidneys in maintaining acid-base balance in the body EXCEPT

(A) the kidneys excrete H^+ ions and form HCO_3^- ions in particular amounts, depending on the acid-base state in the body

(B) when a patient becomes acidotic, serum pH drops and the kidneys excrete H^+ ions and form and retain HCO_3^- ions

(C) when a patient becomes alkalotic, serum pH rises and the kidneys retain H^+ ions and excrete HCO_3^- ions

(D) because the kidneys take only 10 to 20 minutes to respond to an alteration in serum pH, they work very well to stabilize acute acid-base problems in rapidly developing conditions

193. All of the following are parts of the condition known as "compensated" shock EXCEPT

  (A) several body adjustments are made to try to maintain cardiac output and arterial pressure
  (B) the sympathetic nervous system is activated and stimulates the heart to beat stronger and faster to compensate for the decrease in blood flow
  (C) the body diverts blood from non-critical parts such as the skin to maintain perfusion of the brain and other critical organs
  (D) during this stage of shock, the sympathetic nervous system releases acetylcholine to bring about the necessary bodily adjustments

194. "Decompensated" shock has all of the following aspects EXCEPT

  (A) it is also known as progressive shock
  (B) as the cardiovascular system progressively deteriorates, the heart is still able to maintain a normal cardiac output and stable blood pressure
  (C) in this stage, as shock progresses, the perfusion of even critical organs decreases dramatically
  (D) hypotension will develop eventually but is a late sign

195. "Irreversible" shock features all of the following EXCEPT

  (A) rapid deterioration of the cardiovascular system occurs which cannot be reversed by the body or by medical interventions
  (B) during this stage, the body begins to shunt blood away from the brain and the heart to maintain perfusion of the liver and kidneys
  (C) cells in vital organs begin to die from inadequate perfusion
  (D) some of the signs are a marked decrease in responsiveness, decreased respiratory rate, decreased pulse rate, and inability to palpate a pulse

196. All of the following are types of shock EXCEPT

  (A) hypovolemic
  (B) neurogenic
  (C) urologic
  (D) cardiogenic

197. The initial assessment of a patient in shock should include all of the following EXCEPT

  (A) airway
  (B) breathing
  (C) pulse oximetry
  (D) level of consciousness

198. In treating a patient in shock, one considers how to manage the patient's airway. All of the following are parts of airway management in a shock patient EXCEPT

(A) nasopharyngeal or oropharyngeal airway
(B) repeated suctioning of the airway
(C) endotracheal intubation
(D) with recurrent oral secretions, placing the patient in the Trendelenburg's position

199. You arrive at a scene of domestic violence and find a 20-year-old male bleeding from a large knife wound in the left leg. He is in shock with a blood pressure of 50 systolic, is lethargic, and has cool clammy skin. You open his airway and notice that the patient is breathing only six times per minute. Your next immediate step should be to

(A) contact medical control to discuss the case
(B) assist the patient's breathing with a bag-valve-mask
(C) perform a complete head-to-toe secondary assessment
(D) attempt to do basic bloodwork

200. After stabilizing a shock patient's airway and assisting the patient's breathing, when the patient has a blood pressure of 50 systolic, you begin to manage the patient's circulation. All of the following are correct steps EXCEPT

(A) start intravenous (IV) lines
(B) perform venipuncture for basic bloodwork
(C) place the patient in a supine position and elevate his or her legs 10 to 12 inches
(D) place a pneumatic antishock garment and inflate as needed

201. All of the following are contraindications to the inflation of the abdominal compartment of a pneumatic antishock garment (PASG) EXCEPT

(A) pregnancy
(B) an impaled object
(C) evisceration
(D) acute gastrointestinal (GI) bleeding

202. All of the following are indications for the use of a PASG EXCEPT

(A) hypovolemic shock
(B) cardiogenic shock
(C) to splint lower extremity fractures
(D) to control blood loss

203. Which of the following is an absolute contraindication to the use of a PASG?

(A) Pulmonary edema
(B) Pregnancy
(C) Head trauma
(D) Impaled objects

204. You are dispatched to a "GI bleeder." As you arrive at the patient's home, you find a 50-year-old male lying in bed with three large bowls filled with blood. The patient's wife notes that he has been having black bowel movements for 2 days and for the past 6 hours has vomited bright red blood on and off. The patient has a history of stomach ulcers and has been taking 8 to 10 aspirins a day for the past week for low back pain. Your assessment reveals the patient to be very weak and lethargic with cool, clammy skin. His vital signs are a blood pressure of 50 palpable systolic, a pulse of 140 per minute and regular, and breathing at 32 breaths per minute. Since you suspect that the patient is in hemorrhagic shock, you apply a 100% oxygen non-rebreather face mask and elevate the patient's legs 10 to 12 inches. Your partner is beginning to set up two intravenous lines. He calls out to ask you what solutions should be set up for those lines. Which is the best choice of solutions for the two lines?

(A) Lactated Ringer's solution and a D$_5$W solution
(B) Two lactated Ringer's solutions
(C) Lactated Ringer's solution and a normal saline solution
(D) Normal saline and a D$_5$W solution

205. All of the following are correct statements concerning blood for transfusions EXCEPT

(A) packed red blood cells, whole blood, plasma, and platelets are all blood products that can be transfused into a patient
(B) packed erythrocytes (red blood cells) are erythrocytes which have been separated from plasma
(C) packed red blood cells, whole blood, plasma, and platelets all can restore the oxygen-carrying capacity of the body
(D) plasma is frequently transfused into patients who have suffered severe burns

ASSESSMENT AND MANAGEMENT OF SHOCK

ANSWERS

172. The answer is C. (Mosby, *Assessment and Management of Shock*. Brady, *Fluids and Shock*.) (A), (B), and (D) are correct. (C) is incorrect because it is anaerobic metabolism that results in a buildup of pyruvic acid which degrades to lactic acid.

173. The answer is B. (Mosby, *Assessment and Management of Shock*.) (B) is the best definition. (A), (C), and (D) are incorrect.

174. The answer is C. (Brady, *Fluids and Shock*. Mosby, *Assessment and Management of Shock*.) (A), (B), and (D) are three of the four elements of the Fick principle. (C) is incorrect because the fourth element requires an adequate number of red blood cells (not white blood cells) to carry the oxygen and adequate perfusion.

175. The answer is C. (Mosby, *Assessment and Management of Shock*.) (A), (B), and (D) are incorrect. (C) is correct because under normal circumstances the cardiovascular system is a closed system of blood vessels that work in conjunction with the heart.

176. The answer is D. (Mosby, *Assessment and Management of Shock*.) (A), (B), (C), contractility, blood pressure, and the blood vessels all affect the ability of the heart to function as the lead organ in the cardiovascular system.

177. The answer is A. (Mosby, *Assessment and Management of Shock*.) (B), (C), and (D) are correct. (A) is incorrect because the bronchi and bronchioles are part of the respiratory system, not the cardiovascular system.

178. The answer is A. (Mosby, *Assessment and Management of Shock*.) (B), (C), and (D) are all correct. (A) is incorrect because water is the most abundant substance in the human body.

179. The answer is B. (Mosby, *Assessment and Management of Shock.*) (A), (C), and (D) are correct. (B) is incorrect because the extracellular fluid accounts for 15–20 percent of total body weight and 25 percent of all body fluid. As a result, the extracellular fluid compartment is made up of 4.5 percent intravascular fluid and 10.5 percent interstitial fluid.

180. The answer is D. (Brady, *Fluids and Shock.*) (A), (B), (C), and magnesium are significant cations in the body. Cadmium is not.

181. The answer is C. (A), (B), and (D) are correct. (C) is incorrect because sulfate (SO_4^-) is not a significant anion in the body.

182. The answer is D. (Mosby, *Assessment and Management of Shock.*) (A), (B), and (C) are incorrect. (D) is a correct statement explaining the cell membrane's semipermeable nature.

183. Answers. (Mosby, *Assessment and Management of Shock.*)
  (A) 2
  (B) 3
  (C) 4
  (D) 5
  (E) 1

184. The answer is D. (Mosby, *Assessment and Management of Shock.*) (A), (B), and (C) are correct. (D) is incorrect because 5% saline is a hypertonic solution.

185. Answers. (Mosby, *Assessment and Management of Shock.* Brady, *Fluids and Shock.*)
  (A) 3
  (B) 1
  (C) 4
  (D) 6
  (E) 2
  (F) 5

186. The answer is D. (Mosby, *Assessment and Management of Shock.*) (A), (B), and (C) are correct. (D) is incorrect because type O blood has no surface antigens. Donors with type O blood are known as universal donors.

187. The answer is C. (Mosby, *Assessment and Management of Shock.* Brady, *Fluids and Shock.*) (A), (B), and (D) are correct. Type B blood has anti-A antibodies and will clump in type A blood. (C) is incorrect because type AB blood has no antibodies to type A and type B blood, and persons with type AB can receive blood from most donors.

188. The answer is A. (Mosby, *Assessment and Management of Shock.* Brady, *Fluids and Shock.*) (B), (C), and (D) are correct. (A) is incorrect because 85 percent of persons in the United States are Rh-positive.

189. **The answer is C.** (Mosby, *Assessment and Management of Shock.* Brady, *Fluids and Shock.*) (A), (B), and (D) are correct. (C) is incorrect because the pH of the human body is usually between 7.35 and 7.45.

190. **The answer is A.** (Mosby, *Assessment and Management of Shock.*) (B), (C) and (D) are correct. (A) is incorrect because these buffer systems are fast-acting defenses that provide almost immediate buffering action against changes in hydrogen ion concentration in the extracellular fluid.

191. **The answer is D.** (Mosby, *Assessment and Management of Shock.*) (A), (B), and (C) are all correct. (D) is incorrect because patients with metabolic acidosis, such as diabetic ketoacidosis, traumatic shock, and aspirin ingestion, compensate by hyperventilating to decrease carbon dioxide and thus decrease the acidosis.

192. **The answer is D.** (Mosby, *Assessment and Management of Shock.*) (A), (B), and (C) are correct. (D) is incorrect because the kidneys take at least 10 to 20 hours (not minutes) to respond to an alteration in serum pH. The kidneys are excellent at long-term compensation but not for acute, rapidly developing conditions.

193. **The answer is D.** (Mosby, *Assessment and Management of Shock.* Brady, *Fluids and Shock.*) (A), (B), and (C) are correct. (D) is incorrect because sympathetic stimulation causes the release of epinephrine from the adrenals and norepinephrine from nerve endings.

194. **The answer is B.** (Mosby, *Assessment and Management of Shock.* Brady, *Fluids and Shock.*) (A), (C), and (D) are correct. (B) is incorrect because as the cardiovascular system deteriorates, cardiac output falls dramatically and leads to further drops in blood pressure.

195. **The answer is B.** (Mosby, *Assessment and Management of Shock.* Brady, *Fluids and Shock.*) (A), (C), and (D) are all correct. (B) is incorrect because in the "irreversible" stage of shock, the body shunts blood away from the kidneys, lungs, and liver to maintain perfusion of the brain and heart.

196. **The answer is C.** (Mosby, *Assessment and Management of Shock.* Brady, *Fluids and Shock.*) (A), (B), (D), septic shock, and anaphylactic shock are five forms of shock. (C) is incorrect because there is no such condition as urologic shock.

197. **The answer is C.** (Mosby, *Assessment and Management of Shock.* Brady, *Fluids and Shock.*) Airway, breathing, circulation, level of consciousness (which represents disability), and exposing the patient are all part of the assessment of a patient in shock.

198. **The answer is D.** (Mosby, *Assessment and Management of Shock.*) (A), (B), (C), and esophageal obturator airway are parts of the management of a shock patient's airway. (D) is incorrect because a shock patient with recurrent secretions should be placed on his or her side, not in the Trendelenburg's position.

199. **The answer is B.** (Mosby, *Assessment and Management of Shock.*) The first management priorities in a shock patient are (A) airway, (B) breathing, (C) circulation, (D) disability, and (E) exposing the patient. Since the airway has been established and secured and the patient is hypoventilating, the next priority is to assist the patient's breathing. Therefore, (B) is the correct answer.

200. **The answer is B.** (Mosby, *Assessment and Management of Shock.*) (A), (C), and (D) are correct. (B) is incorrect because in the prehospital setting, doing basic bloodwork is not a priority. It will be performed at arrival in the emergency department.

201. **The answer is D.** (Mosby, *Assessment and Management of Shock.* Brady, *Fluids and Shock.*) (A), (B), (C), and respiratory distress are contraindications to the inflation of the abdominal compartment of a PASG. (D) is incorrect because bleeding, including acute GI bleeding, is a common indication for the use of a PASG.

202. **The answer is B.** (Mosby, *Assessment and Management of Shock.* Brady, *Fluids and Shock.*) (A), (C), and (D) are correct. (B) is incorrect because cardiogenic shock, which includes pulmonary edema, is a contraindication to the use of a PASG.

203. **The answer is A.** (Mosby, *Assessment and Management of Shock.* Brady, *Fluids and Shock.*) (A) is an absolute contraindication. Many authorities also consider penetrating neck and/or chest trauma as an absolute contraindication. (B) and (D) are relative contraindications because one may inflate the leg compartments but not the abdominal compartment. (C) is a contraindication only if the systolic blood pressure is above 100 because inflation of the PASG may increase intracranial pressure.

204. **The answer is C.** (Mosby, *Assessment and Management of Shock.* Brady, *Fluids and Shock.*) (C) is correct because both are isotonic crystalloid solutions which will produce an immediate expansion of the patient's circulatory system. While (B) would produce the same immediate expansion, it is preferable to have at least one intravenous line of normal saline because it is acceptable for receiving whole blood and packed red blood cell transfusions, which would be given in the emergency department. Lactated Ringer's solution is not compatible with blood transfusions. (A) and (D) are incorrect because D_5W is a hypotonic solution and plays no role in the treatment of hemorrhagic shock.

205. **The answer is C.** (Mosby, *Assessment and Management of Shock.*) (A), (B), and (D) are correct. (C) is incorrect because only the infusion of erythrocytes (red blood cells) in the form of packed erythrocytes or whole blood is capable of restoring the oxygen-carrying capacity of the body. Plasma and platelets cannot do this.

INTRAVENOUS CANNULATION

In this chapter, you will review:

- indications and contraindications
- venous access
- problematic intravenous lines

INTRAVENOUS CANNULATION

Directions: Each item below contains four suggested responses. Select the **one best** response to each item.

206. Which of the following is the correct definition of *intravenous cannulation*?

(A) Pushing medication into a vein
(B) Performing an arterial blood gas
(C) Placing a catheter into a vein
(D) Measuring the pressure in a vein

207. All of the following are indications for performing intravenous (IV) cannulation EXCEPT

(A) hypoglycemia
(B) heart disease
(C) seizure
(D) headache

208. All of the following are contra-indications to performing intravenous cannulation EXCEPT

(A) patients less than 5 or more than 80 years of age
(B) a burned extremity
(C) a sclerotic vein
(D) delaying the transport of a critically ill or injured patient

209. All of the following are used to perform intravenous cannulation EXCEPT

(A) IV solution, administration kit, extension set
(B) needles/catheters, gloves, tourniquet
(C) IV antibiotics, blood products
(D) tape, gauze dressings, padded armboards

210. All of the following are correct statements concerning the use of 5% dextrose in water (D_5W) as an intravenous solution EXCEPT

(A) it is the solution of choice for the treatment of shock
(B) it will maintain water balance and supply calories for cell metabolism
(C) it is a hypotonic sugar solution
(D) it may cause hyponatremia, hyperglycemia, and water intoxication

211. All of the following are correct statements about the use of lactated Ringer's solution EXCEPT

(A) it contains sodium chloride, potassium chloride, calcium chloride, and sodium lactate in water
(B) it is an isotonic crystalloid solution
(C) it can be administered aggressively to patients with congestive heart failure (CHF) and/or pulmonary edema
(D) it is used frequently in the treatment of shock

212. All of the following are correct statements concerning the use of 0.9% sodium chloride solution (normal saline) as an intravenous solution EXCEPT

(A) it is an isotonic solution
(B) it is used frequently in patients with shock
(C) it contains sodium, potassium, glucose, and chloride
(D) it is used with caution in patients with CHF or renal dysfunction

213. Colloid solutions are characterized by all of the following EXCEPT

(A) they contain large molecules which remain in the intravascular space
(B) examples are whole blood, packed red blood cells, plasma, and dextran
(C) they are used frequently in the prehospital setting
(D) they are called volume expanders

214. You respond to a "stabbing." As you arrive in the apartment, you are told that there was an argument and that the wife used a kitchen knife to slash her husband on the neck after she was hit several times. There is a pool of blood (about 500 mL) next to the patient, who is lethargic on the floor. The patient's blood pressure is palpable at 50, and his pulse is 140 per minute. He is cool and clammy as well. Your partner started an IV with lactated Ringer's. You both recall the correct ratio of IV crystalloid solution to every liter of blood loss. Which of the following is the correct ratio?

(A) 1:1 ratio, 500 mL in this case
(B) 2:1 ratio, 1000 mL in this case
(C) 3:1 ratio, 1500 mL in this case
(D) 4:1 ratio, 2000 mL in this case

215. The correct IV flow rate is determined by the patient's response to treatment. All of the following are signs of an improving response to a given IV flow rate EXCEPT

(A) pulse
(B) blood pressure
(C) capillary response
(D) temperature

216. All of the following are true advantages, disadvantages, or complications with the use of metacarpal veins located on the dorsum of the hand EXCEPT

(A) they are easily accessible
(B) with hypovolemia, peripheral veins are the best access sites
(C) the EMT-I should be allowed to start successive venipuncture above the previous puncture site
(D) this site becomes phlebitic easily

217. All of the following are true advantages, disadvantages, or complications with the use of the cephalic vein, which is located along the radial side of the forearm and upper arm EXCEPT

(A) it is a small vein that is difficult to cannulate
(B) it accepts large-bore needles
(C) it tends to roll during needle insertion
(D) its position on the forearm creates a natural splint for the needle and adapter

218. All of the following are true advantages, disadvantages, or complications with the use of the antecubital veins EXCEPT

(A) the median cubital vein is located in front of the elbow
(B) they are readily accessible large veins
(C) they cannot be used in children
(D) it is difficult to splint the area, and with elbow joint flexion any movement can dislodge the catheter and cause infiltration or phlebitis

219. All of the following are true advantages, disadvantages, or complications with the use of the external jugular vein EXCEPT

(A) it is considered a central vein
(B) it is easy to cannulate
(C) it provides rapid access to the central circulation
(D) during cardiac arrest it may not be readily available to the EMT-Intermediate (EMT-I) because the partner is working to manage the airway

220. All of the following veins are commonly used for peripheral intravenous cannulation. Match these commonly used veins with the correct anatomic locations:

(A) Digital veins _____
(B) Metacarpal veins _____
(C) Cephalic vein _____
(D) Basilic vein _____
(E) Antecubital vein _____
(F) Great saphenous vein _____
(G) External jugular vein _____

1. Located at internal malleolus of the ankle
2. Dorsum of the hand
3. Lateral and dorsum of the fingers
4. Runs along the radial side of forearm and upper arm
5. Located in the antecubital fossa
6. Runs behind the angle of the jaw
7. Ascends along the ulnar side of the forearm and upper arm

221. All of the following are steps involved in performing peripheral venous cannulation EXCEPT

(A) explain the procedure and the need for it to the patient
(B) select and check the IV fluid, the appropriate-size catheter, and the administration set
(C) find the appropriate vein, cleanse the site with iodine or an alcohol wipe, and apply the tourniquet
(D) perform the venipuncture and draw a blood sample while leaving the tourniquet in place

222. All of the following are questions relating to IVs that are not functioning properly EXCEPT

(A) was the tourniquet removed?
(B) is there swelling at the cannulation site?
(C) is the flow regulator in the open position?
(D) is the IV cannulation site high enough for the IV bag?

223. All of the following are complications of intravenous therapy EXCEPT

(A) extravasation and hematoma
(B) seizures and migraine headaches
(C) thrombophlebitis and catheter shear
(D) air embolism and arterial puncture

224. All of the following are steps taken in removing an intravenous line EXCEPT

(A) use rubber gloves, sterile gauze, and tape
(B) after carefully untaping, remove the dressing
(C) withdraw the intravenous catheter by pulling straight back, then cover with a sterile dressing and hold against the puncture site until the bleeding stops
(D) after doing all of the above, close the IV flow control valve completely

INTRAVENOUS CANNULATION

ANSWERS

206. The answer is C. (Mosby, *IV Cannulation.*) (C) is correct. This procedure is performed to administer blood, fluids, or medications directly into the circulatory system. (A), (B), and (D) are all incorrect.

207. The answer is D. (Mosby, *IV Cannulation.*) (A), (B), (C), hypovolemia, shock, and a need for IV access to administer medication are some of the more common indications for intravenous cannulation. (D) is incorrect because a headache is not by itself an indication for intravenous cannulation.

208. The answer is A. (Mosby, *IV Cannulation.*) (B) and (C) are contraindications; however, one still can perform intravenous cannulation at another site, such as the other nonburned extremity. (D) is also a contraindication. The local medical direction often has guidelines for performing intravenous cannulation on critically ill or injured patients. Sometimes scoop and run is recommended; others recommend performing intravenous cannulation while in transport or set a limit on the number of attempts (one or two before transport). (A) is incorrect because there are no age limits for performing intravenous cannulation. The local medical direction may set pediatric guidelines.

209. The answer is C. (Mosby, *IV Cannulation.*) (A), (B), (D), 10- to 35-mL syringes, vacu-tainers, blood collection tubes, gowns and goggles, and antibiotic swabs and ointment are the types of equipment used to perform IV cannulation. (C) is incorrect because while IV antibiotics and blood products frequently are administered intravenously, they are not considered part of the equipment needed to perform intravenous cannulation.

210. The answer is A. (Mosby, *IV Cannulation.* Brady, *Fluids and Shock.*) (B), (C), and (D) are correct. (A) is incorrect because 5 percent dextrose in water (D_5W) is not the solution of choice for the treatment of shock. Depending on the medical control, lactated Ringer's solution and/or 0.9 percent sodium chloride solution (normal saline) are the solutions of choice for the treatment of shock.

211. The answer is C. (Mosby, *IV Cannulation.* Brady, *Fluids and Shock.*) (A), (B), and (D) are correct. (C) is incorrect because one must use lactated Ringer's solution cautiously in a patient with CHF or pulmonary edema. It may actually precipitate CHF or pulmonary edema in certain patients.

212. The answer is C. (Mosby, *IV Cannulation.* Brady, *Fluids and Shock.*) (A), (B), and (D) are correct. (C) is incorrect because normal saline contains sodium and chloride in water. It does not contain potassium and glucose.

213. The answer is C. (Mosby, *IV Cannulation.* Brady, *Fluids and Shock.*) (A), (B), and (D) are correct. (C) is incorrect because colloid solutions require special storage, are expensive, and are used infrequently in the prehospital setting.

214. The answer is C. (Mosby, *IV Cannulation.*) The correct ratio of IV crystalloid to every liter of blood loss is 3:1.

215. The answer is D. (Mosby, *IV Cannulation.*) (A), (B), (C), and cerebral function are clinical signs for monitoring the response to a given IV flow rate. (D) is incorrect because it is not related to the IV flow rate.

216. The answer is B. (Mosby, *IV Cannulation.*) (A), (C), and (D) are true. (B) is incorrect because in a hypovolemic patient the peripheral veins collapse more readily than do the large veins.

217. The answer is A. (Mosby, *IV Cannulation.*) (B), (C), and (D) are correct. (A) is incorrect because the cephalic vein is a large vein which is excellent for venipuncture.

218. The answer is C. (Mosby, *IV Cannulation.*) (A), (B), and (D) are correct. (C) is incorrect because the antecubital veins are often visible or palpable in children.

219. The answer is A. (Mosby, *IV Cannulation.*) (B), (C), and (D) are correct. (A) is incorrect because while the external jugular vein does provide rapid access to the central circulation, it is still considered a peripheral vein.

220. Answers.
    (A) 3
    (B) 2
    (C) 4
    (D) 7
    (E) 5
    (F) 1
    (G) 6

221. **The answer is C.** (Mosby, *IV Cannulation.*) (A), (B), and (D) are correct. (C) is incorrect because the EMT-I should apply the tourniquet, then find the appropriate vein, and then cleanse the site with iodine or an alcohol wipe.

222. **The answer is D.** (Mosby, *IV Cannulation.*) (A), (B), and (C) are correct. (D) is incorrect because the IV bag must be high enough for gravity to move the IV fluid through the IV cannulation site.

223. **The answer is B.** (Mosby, *IV Cannulation.* Brady, *Fluids and Shock.*) (A), (C), (D), a pyrogenic reaction, and pain are all complications of intravenous therapy. (B) is incorrect because seizures and migraines are not related to intravenous therapy.

224. **The answer is D.** (Mosby, *IV Cannulation.*) (A), (B), and (C) are correct. (D) is incorrect because the IV flow control valve should be closed before performing step (B).

PHARMACOLOGY

In this chapter, you will review:

- dosage calculations

- appropriate techniques for drug administration

- primary drugs administered by EMT-I

PHARMACOLOGY

Directions: Each item below contains four suggested responses. Select the **one best** response to each item.

225. Which of the following is the BEST definition of a drug?

    (A) A medication which is ingested only and results in sedation

    (B) A chemical product which is created by a pharmacy and is available only by prescription

    (C) A substance taken into the body which changes one or more bodily functions

    (D) A particular substance that causes damage to certain organs

226. Which of the following is the BEST definition of pharmacology?

    (A) A company which produces numerous drugs

    (B) A professional who prepares medications and distributes them by prescription from a physician

    (C) The study of the normal functions of the organs of the body

    (D) The study of drugs and their actions, doses, and side effects

227. All of the following are names given to a drug EXCEPT

    (A) chemical name
    (B) formulary name
    (C) trade name
    (D) generic name

228. Match the following laws which regulate drugs with the correct descriptions:

(A) Harrison Narcotic Act _____
(B) Narcotic Control Act _____
(C) Federal Food, Drug and Cosmetic Act _____
(D) Pure Food and Drug Act _____
(E) Controlled Substances Act _____

1. Passed in 1906; prevents the manufacture of and trafficking in mislabeled, poisonous, or harmful foods and drugs
2. Passed in 1914; the first federal legislation to combat drug addiction or dependency
3. Passed in 1970; regulates the manufacture and distribution of drugs which may cause dependency
4. Passed in 1956; makes the possession of heroin and marijuana illegal
5. Passed in 1939; requires that labels be used to list habit-forming properties and side effects

229. Match the following five schedules of drugs established by the Drug Enforcement Agency with the correct definition:

(A) Schedule I _____
(B) Schedule II _____
(C) Schedule III _____
(D) Schedule IV _____
(E) Schedule V _____

1. Drugs with the highest abuse potential and currently not acceptable for medical use in the United States
2. Drugs that have a lower potential for abuse and are used for coughs or diarrhea and contain limited amounts of narcotics, such as paregoric
3. Drugs with a limited potential for psychological and physiologic dependence, such as paregoric, fiorinal, and Tylenol with codeine
4. Drugs with high potential for abuse that require a written prescription and cannot be refilled, such as morphine, cocaine, and codeine
5. Drugs with a lower potential for abuse that can be called in to the pharmacist, such as Valium, Librium, and phenobarbital

230. All of the following are U.S. drug-regulating agencies EXCEPT

    (A) Federal Communication Commission
    (B) Federal Trade Commission
    (C) Drug Enforcement Administration
    (D) Food and Drug Agency

231. All of the following are drug references available to an EMT-Intermediate (EMT-I) EXCEPT

    (A) *Physicians Desk Reference* (PDR)
    (B) *Glossary of Drugs*
    (C) *Compendium of Drug Therapy*
    (D) *American Hospital Formulary Service*

232. All of the following are sources of drug EXCEPT

    (A) animals
    (B) plants
    (C) laboratory synthesis
    (D) plastics

233. In the prehospital setting, EMT-Is frequently administer parenteral medications subcutaneously, intramuscularly, or intravenously. These drugs are packaged in all of the following forms EXCEPT

    (A) ampuls
    (B) prefilled syringes
    (C) prefilled intravenous tubing
    (D) vials

234. Match the following subjects with the correct definitions:

    (A) Drug action _____
    (B) Drug effect _____
    (C) Pharmacokinetics _____

    1. Movement of drugs through the body; includes absorption, distribution, metabolism, and excretion
    2. Cellular change effected by a drug
    3. Degree of the physiologic change caused by a drug

235. All of the following are factors which affect the actions of drugs on the body EXCEPT

    (A) age
    (B) weight
    (C) IQ
    (D) tolerance

236. All of the following are true statements concerning the sympathetic division of the autonomic nervous system EXCEPT

    (A) two types of sympathetic nerve receptors are alpha-adrenergic and beta-adrenergic (beta$_1$ and beta$_2$)
    (B) the primary effect of sympathetic stimulation is decreased heart rate, bronchoconstriction, and decreased metabolism and strength
    (C) after sympathetic nerve stimulation, an impulse is carried across a synapse (nerve junction) by a chemical transmitter known as norepinephrine
    (D) drugs that stimulate the sympathetic nerve are called alpha-adrenergic and/or beta-adrenergic agonists

237. All of the following are true statements concerning the parasympathetic division of the autonomic nervous system EXCEPT

(A) after parasympathetic nerve stimulation, a message is carried across the synapse by the primary parasympathetic neurotransmitter, which is known as acetylcholine

(B) the seventh cranial nerve, the facial nerve, is the primary nerve of the parasympathetic division and accounts for 75 percent of its actions

(C) acetylcholine is finally broken down by the enzyme cholinesterase

(D) the primary effect of parasympathetic stimulation is decreased heart rate and increased activity in the stomach and gastrointestinal tract for digestion

238. You are dispatched to a 5-year-old boy found in the garage with a possible overdose. As you approach the child, his parents are frantic, stating that he was left playing in the basement but then wandered into the garage. The child is unconscious, and an open bottle of insecticide is lying next to him On inspection, his pupils are pinpoint, he is salivating, his eyes are tearing, and he is cyanotic with a tight chest (poor air exchange), muscle twitching, and a heart rate of 32 per minute. You can see that the child has had urinary and rectal incontinence. All of the following are true concerning this insecticide overdose EXCEPT

(A) the antidote of choice is epinephrine

(B) the tremendous parasympathetic outflow from an insecticide overdose is due to an inhibition of cholinesterase, which prevents the breakdown of acetylcholine

(C) insecticide poisoning is also known as organophosphate poisoning

(D) certain medications also inhibit cholinesterase, for example, physostigmine, neostigmine, and edrophonium

239. All of the following are examples of the correct use of decimals EXCEPT

(A) 8/100 = 0.08
(B) 0.74 − 0.52 = 0.22
(C) 0.82 × .4 = 0.328
(D) 7.765 is rounded off to 7.76

240. You are dispatched to a cardiac patient who is complaining of palpitations. The patient denies chest pain or shortness of breath but admits to a rapid heartbeat associated with weakness and dizziness. On physical examination, his blood pressure is 70/50 with a pulse of 180 per minute, with the remainder of the examination being unremarkable. Your cardiac monitor shows ventricular tachycardia. As you send the rhythm strip to the Emergency Department physician, you ask to give a bolus dose of intravenous lidocaine. The patient states that he weighs 176 lb, and the physician requests a bolus of 1 mg/kg. You have a prefilled 10-mL syringe with a concentration of 10 mg/mL. Which of the following is the correct dose and amount to administer?

(A) A 176-mg dose by giving 17.6 mL of a prefilled syringe
(B) A 17.6-mg dose by giving 1.76 mL of a prefilled syringe
(C) An 8-mg dose by giving 0.8 mL of a prefilled syringe
(D) An 80-mg dose by giving 8 mL of a prefilled syringe

241. You are dispatched to a baby in cardiac arrest at home. As you arrive, the child's father leads you to the infant's room, where the mother is performing cardiopulmonary resuscitation (CPR). The father states that the child has had a little cold for the past 2 days. However, when the baby did not cry during the night, the mother went in to check and found him unresponsive, cold, and not breathing. As your partner gently takes over the care, he confirms that the 2-month-old baby is truly in cardiac arrest. As he continues CPR, you set up for and perform endotracheal intubation. According to your pediatric protocols, the next step is to administer endotracheal epinephrine. The mother states that the child weighs 13.5 lb. Your protocol states that you are to administer 0.1 mg/kg, and you have a 10-mL prefilled syringe of a 1:10,000 solution with a concentration of 0.1 mg/mL. Which of the following is the correct dose and amount to administer?

(A) 13.5 mg, 13.5 mL of the 1:10,000 solution
(B) 8.0 mg, 8.0 mL of the 1:10,000 solution
(C) 0.6 mg, 6.0 mL of the 1:10,000 solution
(D) 6.0 mg, 6.0 mL of the 1:10,000 solution

242. You respond to an 80-year-old man who has just passed out. The patient states that he was walking to the grocery store and only remembers awakening with a group of people around him. He denies any focal pain from the fall. As you begin to examine the patient, you notice that he is in no acute distress. His vital signs are a blood pressure of 100/68, respirations of 14 per minute, and a pulse of 30 per minute. Upon further questioning, the patient denies chest pain, shortness of breath, headache, focal weakness, previous syncopal episodes, or taking any cardiac medications. As you attach the patient to a cardiac monitor, you note that he is in third-degree heart block with a ventricular rate of 24 per minute. A repeat blood pressure is 90/60. You call medical control to request permission to administer intravenous (IV) atropine. The patient states that he weighs 110 lb. Your protocol states that the dose is 0.5 to 1.0 mg every 3–5 minutes to a maximum 0.04 mg/kg, and you have a 10-mL prefilled syringe of 0.1 mg/mL. Which item lists the maximal dose and the maximal amount to administer?

(A) 2.0 mg, 10 mL
(B) 3.0 mg, 10 mL
(C) 2.0 mg, 20 mL
(D) 3.0 mg, 20 mL

243. Match each drug route with the correct indication, description, or particular example:
(A) Sublingual _____
(B) Subcutaneous _____
(C) Intraosseous _____
(D) Transdermal _____
(E) Inhalation _____
(F) Intravenous _____
(G) Endotracheal _____
(H) Intramuscular _____

1. Absorption through the skin
2. In cardiac arrest, an EMT-I may administer certain drugs
3. Nitroglycerin: EMT-B may assist patient to administer
4. Small quantities of drug administered
5. Quickest entry into bloodstream
6. Rapid vascular access for a critically injured child
7. Route for drugs not to be absorbed as quickly as intramuscular or IV
8. Drug quickly absorbed through alveolar walls into capillaries

244. Match each administration device with the correct characteristic or indication for a particular drug:

(A) 3-mL hypodermic needle _____

(B) 25-gauge, ⅝-inch or 23-gauge, ½-inch needle _____

(C) Total capacity of 1 mL with 100 calibration lines (0.01 mL each) _____

(D) Total 1 mL, each 10 units divided by five small lines _____

(E) Prefilled syringe _____

1. Insulin syringe
2. Used for subcutaneous injections
3. Tuberculin syringe
4. Most commonly used syringe
5. Contains premeasured amount of medication

245. As an EMT-I, you consider the techniques used to administer drugs which are packaged in vials, ampuls, and prefilled syringes. All of the following are steps used to administer medications from vials, ampuls and prefilled syringes EXCEPT

(A) confirm the drug type, concentration, and dose

(B) check the cloudiness and expiration date

(C) place a gauze or alcohol wipe over the neck and snap the top off

(D) invert the syringe and expel any air

246. You are assigned to a 54-year-old male with chest pain. As you arrive at the patient's job site, you find him sitting on a chair and complaining of substernal chest pain associated with sweating and mild shortness of breath. His vital signs and physical examination are grossly normal. You prepare to administer sublingual nitroglycerin. All of the following are parts of the technique used to do this EXCEPT

(A) contact medical control for permission to administer the medication or follow off-line standing orders

(B) check the name, dose, and expiration date

(C) uncap the container and remove the indicated tablet

(D) simply hand the medication to the patient to self-administer orally

247. As an EMT-I, you consider the technique used to administer drugs by the subcutaneous, intramuscular, and intravenous routes. All of the following are steps used for all these routes EXCEPT

(A) use body substance isolation precautions

(B) reassure the patient and check for allergies

(C) after inserting the needle, pull back the syringe plunger; if blood is seen in the syringe, withdraw the needle, apply pressure over the site, and select another site

(D) do not recap the needle

248. You respond to a 28-year-old male overdose patient who is having difficulty breathing. Upon arrival, you find the patient breathing six times a minute with pinpoint pupils and new needle marks on his left arm. Your protocol allows you, by written standing orders, to administer IV Narcan, but you are unable to find a vein, and the patient is now breathing two to three times per minute. After intubating the patient, you prepare to administer Narcan by endotracheal tube. All of the following are parts of the technique for administering Narcan by endotracheal tube EXCEPT

(A) oxygenate and ventilate the patient
(B) hyperventilate the patient
(C) take an initial dose of 2 mg and dilute with normal saline to a volume of 10 mL
(D) follow the administration of the Narcan by the endotracheal tube by giving several positive-pressure ventilations

249. Which of the following is part of the technique used to administer albuterol sulfate to an asthmatic patient?

(A) In preparing an adult dose, begin with 5.0 mg of albuterol sulfate
(B) Confirm the indications for its use: asthma and foreign body airway obstruction
(C) Since it is a fairly benign drug, permission from medical control to administer it is not required
(D) If the patient's bronchospasm is severe, the administration of another drug by another route should be considered

250. Match each drug with the correct indication:

(A) Lidocaine _____
(B) Atropine _____
(C) Naloxone _____
(D) Dextrose 50% solution _____
(E) Albuterol sulfate _____
(F) Epinephrine _____
(G) Nitroglycerin _____

1. Bronchospasm from asthma or emphysema
2. Cardiac arrest, ventricular fibrillation/ventricular tachycardia (VF/VT), wide-complex tachycardia, significant ventricular ectopy
3. Hypoglycemia, altered mental status
4. Cardiac arrest, VF/VT, acute bronchospasm
5. Symptomatic bradycardia
6. Narcotic overdose, altered mental status
7. Angina, congestive heart failure

251. Match each drug with the correct dose and administration route:

(A) Atropine _____

(B) Lidocaine _____

(C) Epinephrine _____

(D) Nitroglycerin _____

(E) Albuterol sulfate _____

(F) Dextrose 50% _____

(G) Naloxone _____

1. Adult dose 0.3–0.4 mg sublingual (SQ); routes: sublingual, transdermal, IV, aerosol

2. Pediatric dose 0.02 mg/kg; routes: IV, IO, ET

3. Adult dose 2.5 mg; route: nebulized inhaler

4. Initial adult dose for cardiac arrest (VF/VT) 1.0–1.5 mg/kg; routes: IV, ET

5. Adult dose 25–50 g; route: IV

6. Pediatric dose ≤ 5 years ≤ 20 kg, 0.1 mg/kg; routes: IV, ET

7. Pediatric dose for bradycardia 0.01 mg/kg IV or 0.1 mg/kg ET; routes: cardiac-related IV, ET, IO and bronchospasm SQ, intramuscular, IV, ET

PHARMACOLOGY

A N S W E R S

225. The answer is C. (Mosby, *Pharmacology.*) (C) is correct. A drug can be created in many locations and is available both by prescription and by illegal means. Every drug changes one or more bodily functions and many of these are positive effects. (A) is incorrect because a drug can enter the body in various ways: orally, sublingually, intramuscularly, transcutaneously, and rectally. A drug can have several effects in addition to sedation.

226. The answer is D. (Mosby, *Pharmacology.*) (D) is correct. (A) is incorrect since it refers to a pharmacy. (B) is incorrect since it refers to a pharmacist. (C) is incorrect since this study is known as pharmaceutical physiology.

227. The answer is B. (Mosby, *Pharmacology.*) (A), (C), (D), and the official name are the four names given to a drug. (B) is incorrect because a formulary is a listing of various drugs, usually by generic and/or trade name. There is no such thing as a drug's formulary name.

228. Answers. (Mosby, *Pharmacology.*)
   (A) 2
   (B) 4
   (C) 5
   (D) 1
   (E) 3

229. Answers. (Mosby, *Pharmacology.*)
   (A) 1
   (B) 4
   (C) 3
   (D) 5
   (E) 2

230. The answer is A. (Mosby, *Pharmacology.*) (B), (C), (D), and the Public Health Service are all drug-regulating agencies. The Federal Communication Commission has nothing to do with drug regulation.

231. The answer is B. (Mosby, *Pharmacology.*) (A), (C), (D), and the *United States Pharmacopeia* (USP) are all references for an EMT-I. (B) is incorrect because there is no such drug reference.

232. The answer is D. (Mosby, *Pharmacology.*) (A), (B), (C), humans, and minerals are all sources of drugs. Plastics are not a source of drugs.

233. The answer is C. (Mosby, *Pharmacology.*) (A), (B), and (D) are correct. (C) is incorrect because this is not a method of packaging parenteral medications.

234. Answers.
(A) 2
(B) 3
(C) 1

235. The answer is C. (Mosby, *Pharmacology.*) (A), (B), (D), gender, and existing pathology are all factors. (C) is incorrect because a patient's IQ has no influence on the actions of drugs.

236. The answer is B. (Mosby, *Pharmacology.*) (A), (C), and (D) are correct. (B) is incorrect because the primary effect of sympathetic stimulation, (the fight-or-flight response) is increased heart rate, bronchodilation, and increased metabolism and strength.

237. The answer is B. (Mosby, *Pharmacology.*) (A), (C), and (D) are correct. (B) is incorrect because the tenth cranial nerve, the vagus nerve, is the primary nerve of the parasympathetic division and accounts for 75 percent of its actions.

238. The answer is A. (Mosby, *Pharmacology.*) (B), (C), and (D) are all correct. (A) is incorrect because in this case the antidote of choice to combat the parasympathetic excess is atropine. Also, this clinical presentation is the same as that of nerve gas, whose actions are due to its being a cholinesterase inhibitor as well.

239. The answer is D. (Mosby, *Pharmacology.*) (A), (B), and (C) show the correct use of decimals. (D) is incorrect because 7.765 is rounded off to 7.77.

240. The answer is D. (Mosby, *Pharmacology.*) (D) is correct because
Step 1. Calculate the patient's weight in kilograms:
Weight/176 lb = 1 kg/2.2 lb
= 176
= 80 kg

Step 2. Calculate the amount of the dose:

Dose/80 kg = 1.0 mg/1.0 kg = 80 mg

Step 3. Calculate the volume of the dose by using the volume calculation formula:

Volume to administer = dose desired × volume on hand/dose on hand

= 80 mg × 10 mL/100 mg = 8 mL

241. The answer is C. (Mosby, *Pharmacology.*) (C) is correct because

Step 1. Calculate the patient's weight in kilograms:

Weight/13.5 lb = 1 kg/2.2 lb

= 13.5

= 6 kg

Step 2. Calculate the amount of the dose:

Dose/6 kg = 0.1 mg/1.0 kg = 0.6 mg

Step 3. Calculate the volume of the dose by using the volume calculation formula:

Volume to administer = Dose desired × volume on hand/dose on hand

= 0.6 mg × 10 mL/1.0 mg = 6 mL

242. The answer is C. (Mosby, *Pharmacology.*) (C) is correct because

Step 1. Calculate the patient's weight in kilograms:

Weight/110 lb = 1 kg/2.2 lb

= 110

= 50 kg

Step 2. Calculate the amount of the total maximum dose:

Dose/50 kg = 0.04 mg/1.0 kg = 2.0 mg

Step 3. Calculate the volume of the dose by using the volume calculation formula:

Volume to administer = dose desired × volume on hand/dose on hand

= 2.0 mg × 10 mL/1 mg = 20 mL

243. Answers. (Mosby, *Pharmacology.*)

(A) 3
(B) 7
(C) 6
(D) 1
(E) 8
(F) 5
(G) 2
(H) 4

244. Answers. (Mosby, *Pharmacology.*)

(A) 4
(B) 2
(C) 3
(D) 1
(E) 5

245. The answer is C. (Mosby, *Pharmacology.*) (A), (B), and (D) are all parts of the technique used to administer drugs packaged in vials, ampuls, and prefilled syringes. (C) is incorrect because snapping the top off is done only to administer drugs packaged in ampuls, not drugs packaged in vials or prefilled syringes.

246. The answer is D. (Mosby, *Pharmacology.*) (A), (B), and (C) are all correct. (D) is incorrect because you must carefully instruct the patient to place the tablet under the tongue so that it does not get chewed or swallowed.

247. The answer is C. (Mosby, *Pharmacology.*) (A), (B), and (D) are all parts of the technique. (C) is incorrect. In administering drugs by the subcutaneous and intramuscular routes, this is the correct technique. However, in administering drugs by the intravenous route, when you pull back on the syringe and blood is seen, you know that you are in the vein and should then administer the medication.

248. The answer is C. (Mosby, *Pharmacology.* (A), (B), and (D) are correct. C is incorrect because the initial dose of Narcan is 2 mg, but it should be diluted with normal saline to a volume of only 3–5 mL.

249. The answer is D. (Mosby, *Pharmacology.* (D) is correct. This also applies if the patient is unable to inhale the medication. (A) is incorrect because the adult dose is 2.5 mg. (B) is incorrect because the indications are asthma and emphysema, not foreign body airway obstruction. (C) is incorrect because you do need medical control permission, directly or by off-line standing orders, to administer the medication.

250. Answers.
(A) 2
(B) 5
(C) 6
(D) 3
(E) 1
(F) 4
(G) 7

251. Answers.
(A) 2
(B) 4
(C) 7
(D) 1
(E) 3
(F) 5
(G) 6

TRAUMA EMERGENCIES

In this chapter, you will review:

- types of trauma

- spinal immobilization techniques

- burns and burn classifications

TRAUMA EMERGENCIES

Directions: Each item below contains four suggested responses. Select the **one best** response to each item.

252. In evaluating a patient with blunt trauma, all of the following are true EXCEPT

(A) blunt trauma is caused by any type of impact trauma that results in two forces: change of speed and compression

(B) blunt trauma to the heart occurs when it is compressed between the sternum and the spine

(C) blunt trauma to the abdomen can cause damage to the lungs and scrotum

(D) blunt trauma to the brain may occur with nonpenetrating head trauma

253. The following are true statements about penetrating trauma EXCEPT

(A) penetrating trauma is defined as some type of noninvasive injury to the body

(B) an example of a low-energy penetrating injury is an injury from a knife

(C) an example of a medium-level penetrating injury is an injury by a handgun

(D) an example of a high-level penetrating injury is an injury by a hunting rifle

254. All of the following are signs associated with a skull fracture EXCEPT

(A) blood or cerebrospinal fluid draining from the ear or nose

(B) raccoon eyes

(C) jaundice

(D) deformity of the skull

255. As you arrive at the scene of a motor vehicle accident, you are directed to a 50-year-old woman who was thrown through the windshield into a tree. She has sustained severe head trauma and is unconscious with a large skull laceration on the forehead. She has unequal pupils with a dilated right pupil. As you begin to immobilize the patient with a cervical collar and long spine board, you begin to notice that her respirations have changed. She has begun to breathe with a pattern of slow, shallow breaths alternating with rapid, deep breaths. In a patient with serious head trauma this breathing pattern is a sign of increased intracranial pressure. This breathing pattern is known as

(A) agonal respirations
(B) Biot's breathing
(C) postictal respirations
(D) Cheyne-Stokes respirations

256. Another sign of increased intracranial pressure is known as Cushing's reflex. All of the following are parts of this reflex EXCEPT

(A) increased blood sugar
(B) increased blood pressure
(C) increased respiratory rate
(D) decreased pulse rate

257. You are flagged down at the scene of a motor vehicle accident. A frantic witness states that an elderly woman was hit by a motorcycle and was thrown headfirst about 10 feet into the side of a parked car. As you begin to assess the patient, you palpate a large area of swelling in the back of the head. The patient is unconscious. You begin to maintain in-line cervical traction and apply the jaw thrust maneuver. Suddenly the patient begins to flex her elbows, wrists, and legs spontaneously. This body posturing is known as

(A) decerebrate posturing
(B) decorticate posturing
(C) focal seizures
(D) hemiplegia

258. Decorticate posturing and decerebrate posturing indicate that a head trauma patient has

(A) an electrolyte imbalance
(B) loss of consciousness
(C) a severe brain injury
(D) an eye injury

259. Hypoperfusion is BEST defined as

(A) a reduced oxygen concentration in the blood
(B) an increase in blood circulating in the body
(C) fluid passing through an organ or part of the body that does not have properly oxygenated blood
(D) a decrease in blood pressure

260. As you arrive at the scene of a motor vehicle accident, a First Responder approaches you with a description of the accident. A witness stated that the car involved in the accident was swerving down this main avenue at about 40 miles per hour. The car went through a red light and hit a telephone pole head-on. The driver broke the windshield with his head. Along with alcohol on his breath, the patient is complaining of neck pain associated with numbness and tingling in both arms and legs. With this presentation, which of the following is the correct mechanism of spinal injury?

(A) Vertical compression
(B) Rotation
(C) Extension
(D) Flexion

261. Immobilization should be performed in all patients suspected of having a spinal injury. Spinal immobilization consists of immobilizing which two areas?

(A) The arms and the body
(B) The pelvis and the body
(C) The neck and the body
(D) The legs and the body

262. You arrive at the emergency department after evaluating and treating a 30-year-old male who has sustained multiple injuries in a motor vehicle accident. The patient's car blew out a tire while speeding down a nearby highway. The car spun out of control until it hit a cement wall. The patient initially hit his head on the driver's side window, with a witness documenting a loss of consciousness for 10 minutes. He also complained of neck pain and a funny sensation in his arms. After you carefully extricate the patient with a manual in-line cervical spine, your partner proceeds to apply a rigid cervical collar and then assists you in applying spinal immobilization. In the emergency department, as soon as you transfer the patient to the stretcher, a surgical resident begins to remove the cervical collar and spinal immobilization after a somewhat cursory exam. All of the following are possible means of persuading the resident to maintain cervical and spinal immobilization until the appropriate x-rays confirm no spinal injury EXCEPT

(A) reemphasize the mechanism of injury in this patient, the loss of consciousness, and the complaint of neck pain
(B) verbally abuse the resident with loud and personal expletives
(C) produce a picture of the automobile to document the extent of car damage
(D) immediately attempt to review the case with the attending physician in charge of the emergency department

263. All of the following are devices used to provide spinal immobilization EXCEPT

   (A) a Kendrick extrication device (KED)
   (B) one-piece and two-piece cervical spine immobilization devices
   (C) a Hare traction splint
   (D) short and long backboards

264. You arrive at the scene of a factory explosion. The police and fire departments have declared the scene safe. As you enter the building and start to assess a patient with multiple injuries, a portion of the ceiling begins to collapse. Assisted by two other EMT-Intermediates (EMT-Is), you recognize that this is an indication to perform which of the following techniques?

   (A) Jaw thrust
   (B) Normal extrication
   (C) Rapid extrication
   (D) Robert Shaw device

265. All of the following are examples of an unsafe scene which requires the use of rapid extrication techniques EXCEPT

   (A) water over the tops of your shoes
   (B) danger of a structure collapse
   (C) presence or threat of a fire
   (D) danger of an explosion

266. All of the following are life-threatening injuries which require rapid extrication EXCEPT

   (A) cardiac or respiratory arrest
   (B) controllable bleeding
   (C) severe shock
   (D) patients with airways that cannot be maintained in the sitting position

267. You go to the scene of a motorcycle accident. A witness states that the motorcycle skidded out of control and that the driver was thrown and landed chest first into the front of a parked car. After opening the airway with a modified jaw thrust maneuver while your partner provides in-line cervical traction, you begin to apply spinal immobilization. As you begin to assess the patient's ventilation, you note that he is having difficulty breathing. As you palpate his right chest, the patient begins to grimace in pain. While you suspect rib fractures, you also wonder if the patient could have a flail chest. Which of the following is the BEST definition of a flail chest?

   (A) Two or more rib fractures with difficulty breathing
   (B) Three or more rib fractures with difficulty breathing
   (C) Two or more rib fractures in two or more places
   (D) Three or more rib fractures in three or more places

268. You are assigned to a stabbing. As you enter the back alley next to an apartment house, you find a 17-year-old boy clutching his left chest. In using body substance isolation precautions, you begin to cut away the patient's blood-stained shirt to examine the wound and assess the injury. The patient has a 2-cm knife wound in about the fourth left intercostal space in the anterior axillary line. As you consider the possibility of a pneumothorax, all of the following are signs or symptoms of it EXCEPT

(A) hemoptysis (coughing up blood)
(B) shortness of breath
(C) pleuritic chest pain
(D) decreased or absent breath sounds

269. You respond to a domestic violence call and find a hysterical teenage boy screaming that his father just shot his mother in the chest. As you begin to assess the patient, you suspect a possible tension pneumothorax. All of the following are "early" signs of a tension pneumothorax EXCEPT

(A) dyspnea
(B) tachypnea
(C) muffled heart sounds
(D) decreased or absent breath sounds

270. All of the following are late signs or symptoms of a tension pneumothorax EXCEPT

(A) distended neck veins
(B) leg edema
(C) tracheal deviation
(D) narrowed pulse pressure

271. Rapid transport to definitive care is defined as which of the following?

(A) Bringing a patient quickly to the hospital to make a definitive diagnosis
(B) Bringing a patient to the hospital having already made a definite diagnosis
(C) Bringing a patient to the hospital to definitely receive care
(D) Bringing a patient to the hospital for specific care to be given to resolve an illness or injury which cannot be treated in the prehospital setting

272. As you respond to a motor vehicle accident, you find a 37-year-old male with a lap seat belt in place complaining of abdominal pain. The other two occupants, in the front seats, are being taken care of by other paramedics and EMT-Is. All of the following are signs and symptoms of abdominal trauma EXCEPT

(A) abdominal pain
(B) abdominal tenderness
(C) abdominal gas
(D) pelvic instability

273. You are dispatched to a patient who has fallen down a flight of stairs. As you enter the home, the patient's husband states that his 8-month-pregnant wife slipped and fell down a flight of 12 stairs and landed on her side. You carefully provide cervical spine in-line traction and complete spinal immobilization, and the initial vital signs are blood pressure 160/84, pulse 110 per minute, and respirations 20 per minute. As you begin to transport the patient on a long board, you recall the correct position for optimizing venous return in a pregnant patient. That position is which of the following?

    (A) Elevating the feet of the long board into a Trendelenburg's position

    (B) Turning the patient on the long board to the right 90°

    (C) Turning the patient on the long board to the left 90°

    (D) Turning the patient on the long board to the left 10–15°

274. You are dispatched to a "man under a train" in a subway station. As you arrive at the platform, you are notified that the scene is safe and the third rail power has been shut off. As you approach the patient, you see that two paramedics and two EMT-Basics (EMT-Bs) are already rendering care to the patient. However, the paramedic requests that you and your partner transport the patient's right amputated (below the knee) leg. All of the following are parts of the care provided to the amputated leg EXCEPT

    (A) wrap the amputated leg in a dry sterile dressing, a dressing moistened by lactated Ringer's, or a normal saline sterile dressing

    (B) place the wrapped amputated leg in a plastic bag

    (C) place the plastic bag on ice

    (D) transport the amputated leg with the patient even if there is a small delay in patient transport to complete preparation of the amputated leg

275. You go to the scene of a fire and are directed to care for a 7-year-old boy who has been burned. The patient is alert and is crying because he was burned in the fire. On initial assessment, the child's airway is patent, and he is breathing normally at 22 breaths per minute. There is no evidence of any soot or burns around or inside his mouth. As you begin to inspect his right arm, you notice redness and spotty blistering from the elbow to the wrist, with the hand having been spared. This burn covers about one-third of the skin on the right arm. Which of the following is the BEST description of this type of burn?

(A) A 3 percent partial-thickness burn
(B) A 5 percent partial-thickness burn
(C) A 1 percent full-thickness burn
(D) A 10 percent superficial burn

276. You are dispatched to the scene of a garage fire. As you arrive, a family member states that a 60-year-old male was putting gasoline into his lawn mower when his cigarette fell into the gasoline, which resulted in a flash of flames and a small fire. The patient's pants caught on fire, and he continued to try to self-extinguish it. After 10 to 15 minutes, one of the neighbor's children saw smoke and called for help. As you begin to assess the patient, you note that his airway is patent, without oral or perioral burns or black sputum, and his vital signs are stable. As you begin to cut away the patient's pants, you note that from below the right knee to the tips of his toes there is very little skin. The actual appearance is dry, leathery, and white with spots of actual fat tissue being visible. The patient states that he has no pain below the right knee. Which of the following is the correct classification of this type of burn?

(A) A 9 percent full-thickness burn
(B) An 18 percent full-thickness burn
(C) A 9 percent partial-thickness burn
(D) An 18 percent partial-thickness burn

277. Which of the following is a correct statement concerning the difference between an open bone injury and a closed bone injury?

- (A) With an open bone injury, the skin is open but there is never a fracture
- (B) With a closed bone injury, the skin is closed but there is always a fracture
- (C) With an open bone injury, the skin is always open; with a closed bone injury, the skin is always closed
- (D) With an open bone injury, the skin is closed but the bone is fractured

278. In treating a partial-thickness burn and a full-thickness burn, all of the following are true EXCEPT

- (A) apply wet dressings on up to 10 percent of the burned body surface
- (B) use high-concentration oxygen and an intravenous (IV) line
- (C) apply dry dressings to at least 90 percent of the burned body surface
- (D) all partial-thickness blisters should be broken open immediately

279. You are dispatched to a jumper. As you drive up, a witness states that a man was painting a billboard, appeared to slip off, and fell about 20 feet. Since the patient is able to respond to questions, you begin to provide complete spinal immobilization. However, you are trying to assess the entire musculoskeletal system to determine the number and extent of bone or joint injuries. All of the following are symptoms or signs of a bone or joint injury EXCEPT

- (A) deformity of the extremity
- (B) pain and tenderness
- (C) full range of motion of a joint
- (D) injury site swelling, discoloration, or bruising

280. You are dispatched to an 82-year-old male who fell down a flight of stairs. As you arrive at the scene, you find the patient moaning and complaining of right hip pain. He is awake and alert, his airway is patent, and you proceed to provide spinal immobilization. As you begin to assess for musculoskeletal injuries, you find that the patient's right lower extremity is shortened and externally rotated and that the patient is unable to lift his leg. All of the following are complications of musculoskeletal trauma EXCEPT

- (A) urinary frequency and dysuria
- (B) postfracture damage to blood vessels, nerves, and muscles
- (C) a decrease in blood flow from a fractured bone compressing a blood vessel
- (D) extremity paralysis caused by spinal cord damage

281. You are assigned to an elderly female who has a broken arm. At the scene, the patient states that she slipped on ice and landed on her right out-stretched arm. Upon assessment, you palpate the distal right forearm and find a very tender, swollen, and slightly angulated area. After applying a splint from above the elbow to below the wrist, you begin to think about the possible complications of the splinting. All of the following are complications of splinting EXCEPT

(A) numbness at or below the splint
(B) cool fingers below the splint
(C) cellulitis of the right leg
(D) muscle and tissue damage under the splint

TRAUMA EMERGENCIES

252. **The answer is C.** (Mosby, *Trauma Emergencies.*) (A), (B), and (D) are correct statements about blunt trauma. (C) is incorrect because blunt trauma to the abdomen can cause damage to the liver, spleen, kidneys, and/or pancreas. The lungs are in the chest, and the scrotum is outside the abdominal cavity.

253. **The answer is A.** (Mosby, *Trauma Emergencies.*) A knife, a needle, and an icepick are all good examples of weapons that cause a low-energy penetrating trauma. Handgun and some rifle wounds are examples of a medium-energy penetrating trauma. A hunting knife and assault weapon wounds are examples of high-energy penetrating trauma. (A) is incorrect because penetrating trauma is defined as an invasive injury to the body in which a cavity is created.

254. **The answer is C.** (Mosby, *Trauma Emergencies.*) (A), (B), (D), a history of head trauma with or without loss of consciousness, an altered level of responsiveness, sluggish or dilated pupils, a penetrating or impaling injury, and Battle's sign are associated with patients who have skull fractures. Jaundice is characterized by yellow skin and sclera of the eyes. It is frequently associated with a myriad of liver and gallbladder diseases. It is not associated with skull fractures.

255. **The answer is D.** (Mosby, *Trauma Emergencies.*) Cheyne-Stokes respirations, as described in the question, often end the slow, shallow breathing sequence with a short apneic episode. Agonal respirations are seen in a patient who is terminally ill and about to die. Biot's breathing is a pattern of breaths of equal depth alternating with abrupt periods of apnea. It is often seen in patients with meningitis. Postictal respirations are seen after a seizure and sometimes are accompanied by a short period of apnea.

256. The answer is A. (Mosby, *Trauma Emergencies.*) (B), (C), and (D) are part of Cushing's reflex. (A) is unrelated to that reflex.

257. The answer is B. (Brady, *General Patient Assessment and Initial Management.*) Decorticate posturing is correct. Decerebrate posturing is defined as extension of the arms and legs as the back bows forcefully. Focal seizures present as localized tonic-clonic contractions. Hemiplegia is the presence of paralysis on one side of the body.

258. The answer is C. (Brady, *General Patient Assessment and Initial Management.*) Decorticate and decerebrate posturing indicate a severe brain injury.

259. The answer is C. (Mosby, *Trauma Emergencies.*) (C) is correct. (A) is the definition of hypoxemia. (B) is unrelated to hypoperfusion. (D) is the definition of hypotension.

260. The answer is D. (Mosby, *Trauma Emergencies.*) In a flexion-induced spinal injury, the supporting ligaments of the posterior spine are abnormally stretched, leading to tears or avulsions of the spinous processes of the vertebrae. (A) is incorrect because a vertical compression-induced spinal injury occurs when a force is directed along the axis of the spine. This usually results from a fall or a heavy object hitting the top of the head. (B) is incorrect because with an acute severe rotation-induced spinal injury, there may be a dislocation of the intervertebral joints and an unstable fracture as well. (C) is incorrect because an extension-induced spinal injury occurs when the head is hyperextended backward. This results in tearing of the ligaments and vertebral instability.

261. The answer is C. (Mosby, *Trauma Emergencies.*) Spinal immobilization is used to prevent movement and additional injury to the vertebrae and spinal cord. (A), (B), and (D) are incorrect.

262. The answer is B. (Mosby, *Trauma Emergencies.*) While this case presentation is not uncommon, engaging in a shouting match with the surgical resident rarely results in a constructive change in patient management. (A), (C), (D), and appealing to the resident's superiors are all options available for you to discuss your legitimate concerns.

263. The answer is C. (Mosby, *Trauma Emergencies.*) (A), (B), and (D) are all devices used to provide spinal immobilization. A Hare traction splint is used to provide traction for a suspected lower extremity fracture.

264. The answer is C. (Mosby, *Trauma Emergencies.*) Rapid extrication is used only when a patient's life is clearly at risk. The jaw thrust is used to open the airway in a patient with a possible cervical spine injury. Normal extrication is used when the scene is safe. A Robert Shaw device is an oxygen-powered demand valve used to ventilate a patient. It is not related to extrication.

265. The answer is A. (Mosby, *Trauma Emergencies.*) (B), (C), (D), and rising water are indications for using rapid extrication techniques. (A) is incorrect because only if the water is rising do you use rapid extrication techniques.

266. The answer is B. (Mosby, *Trauma Emergencies.*) (A), (C), (D), uncontrollable bleeding, and a mechanism of injury which indicates a potential for rapid decompensation require rapid extrication. (B) is incorrect because only uncontrollable bleeding requires rapid removal.

267. The answer is C. (Brady, *General Patient Assessment and Initial Management.*) (C) is the correct definition of a flail chest, which causes paradoxical movement of the chest and greatly reduces air movement. An underlying pulmonary contusion also contributes to poor oxygenation.

268. The answer is A. (Mosby, *Trauma Emergencies.*) (B), (C), and (D) are signs or symptoms of pneumothorax. (A) is incorrect because hemoptysis is not related to pneumothorax.

269. The answer is C. (Mosby, *Trauma Emergencies.*) Dyspnea, tachypnea, and decreased or absent breath sounds are all early signs of a tension pneumothorax. Muffled heart sounds are a sign of pericardial tamponade but are not related to a tension pneumothorax. However, with a tension pneumothorax, the heart may be displaced opposite to the collapsed lung. Therefore, the heart sounds may be heard best in an unusual location, as in left tension pneumothorax (heart sounds heard best in the right chest) and right tension pneumothorax (heart sounds heard best on the far lateral left chest wall, not at the apex).

270. The answer is B. (Mosby, *Trauma Emergencies.*) Distended neck veins, tracheal deviation, narrowed pulse pressure, tympany, and signs of acute hypoxia are all late signs or symptoms of a tension pneumothorax. Leg edema is not related to a tension pneumothorax.

271. The answer is D. (Mosby, *Trauma Emergencies.*) (D) is the correct definition of definitive care provided at the hospital. (A), (B), and (C) are incorrect definitions.

272. The answer is C. (Mosby, *Trauma Emergencies.*) Abdominal pain, abdominal tenderness, pelvic instability, abdominal rigidity, guarding, bruising, bleeding, and evisceration are all signs of abdominal trauma. Abdominal gas is not a sign or symptom of abdominal trauma.

273. The answer is D. (Mosby, *Trauma Emergencies.*) (D) is the correct position. (A), (B), and (C) are incorrect positions.

274. The answer is D. (Mosby, *Trauma Emergencies.*) (A), (B), and (C) are correct. (D) is incorrect because the transport of a critically ill patient should never be delayed to complete the preparation of an amputated part. That part can be transported separately, especially if it has not yet been found.

275. **The answer is A.** (Mosby, *Trauma Emergencies.*) A 3 percent partial-thickness burn is correct because a partial-thickness burn produces pain with red or white skin which is moist and mottled, usually with blisters. The former name for this type of burn was a second-degree burn. Since the arm of an adult or a child represents 9 percent of the body area and this patient's burn covered one-third of the right arm's skin surface, the correct answer is 3 percent.

276. **The answer is A.** (Mosby, *Trauma Emergencies.*) A 9 percent full-thickness burn is the correct answer because of the lack of pain and the appearance of the burn. There is no identifiable reddening of the skin, which would occur with a superficial (first-degree) burn. There is also no evidence of a painful moist, mottled burn with blistering, which would be consistent with a partial-thickness (second-degree) burn. Also, a man's entire leg encompasses 18 percent of the body area. Since this patient's burn extended below the right knee to his toes, accounting for approximately half of the right leg's surface, it is defined as a 9 percent full-thickness burn.

277. **The answer is C.** (Mosby, *Trauma Emergencies.*) (C) is the correct definition of a closed bone injury and an open bone injury. This definition has nothing to do with the presence or absence of a fracture.

278. **The answer is D.** (Mosby, *Trauma Emergencies.*) (A), (B), and (C) are all correct. (D) is incorrect because partial-thickness (second-degree) blisters should not be broken.

279. **The answer is C.** (Mosby, *Trauma Emergencies.*) Deformity of the extremity; pain and tenderness; injury site swelling, discoloration, or bruising; abnormal position of an extremity; guarding; exposed bone ends; and a joint locked into position are all symptoms or signs of a bone or joint injury. (C) is incorrect because the full range of motion of a joint is a normal finding.

280. **The answer is A.** (Mosby, *Trauma Emergencies.*) (B), (C), (D), conversion of a closed fracture to an open fracture, excessive bleeding, and increased pain from the movement of bone ends are all complications of musculoskeletal trauma. (A) is incorrect because urinary frequency and dysuria are signs of a urinary tract infection. While the urologic system can be damaged by musculoskeletal trauma, a urinary tract infection usually is not related to such a trauma.

281. **The answer is C.** (Mosby, *Trauma Emergencies.*) Numbness, cool fingers, muscle and tissue damage, and mottled skin are all possible complications from applying a splint. (C) is a skin infection of the right leg and is not related to splinting the right forearm.

CARDIAC
EMERGENCIES

In this chapter, you will review:

- recognize and treat angina/acute myocardial infarction

- CHF signs and symptoms

- AED indications

CARDIAC EMERGENCIES

Directions: Each item below contains four suggested responses. Select the **one best** response to each item.

282. All of the following are risk factors for cardiac disease, particularly coronary artery disease, EXCEPT

(A) hypertension
(B) cigarette smoking
(C) insomnia
(D) diabetes

283. All of the following are criteria which must be met before administering nitroglycerin tablets or spray EXCEPT

(A) a patient with cardiac chest pain
(B) EMT-Intermediates (EMT-Is) should try to have medical control authorization to assist a patient in administering nitroglycerin tablets or spray
(C) the patient has physician-prescribed sublingual nitro-glycerin tablets or sprays
(D) in some emergency medical systems (EMS), EMT-Is with medical control authorization may initiate nitroglycerin tablets or spray for patients without a physician's prescription

284. All of the following are side effects of sublingual nitroglycerin tablets and spray EXCEPT

(A) oral fungal infection
(B) headache
(C) tingling under the tongue
(D) hypotension

285. You are dispatched to an office building to see a 45-year-old male with chest pain. The patient states that he is a diabetic and a two-pack-a-day smoker for 20 years, on medications for high blood pressure and angina for 10 years, who felt substernal chest pain for about 1 hour. The pain is squeezing and spreads to both arms. He also has been sweating, short of breath, and nauseated. In assisting this patient to administer his prescribed nitroglycerin tablets, all of the following should be done EXCEPT

(A) make sure the systolic blood pressure is above 100
(B) check the expiration date of the nitroglycerin
(C) before administering nitroglycerin spray, shake the container
(D) put on gloves before placing a nitroglycerin tablet or spray under the tongue

286. All of the following are contraindications to administering nitroglycerin EXCEPT

(A) high blood pressure
(B) systolic blood pressure below 100
(C) infants and children
(D) head injury

287. While you are returning home from a gas station, a man in the street frantically waves you down. He states that a neighbor is in the hallway complaining of severe chest pain. As you open the door of the building, you see a 60-year-old woman clutching her chest while sitting on the floor. She is sweating profusely, breathing rapidly, and appearing pale and acutely ill. You begin to obtain a pertinent history, while taking vital signs, administering oxygen, starting an intravenous (IV) line, and hooking up the patient to a cardiac monitor. In trying to determine whether this patient is having an acute myocardial infarction (MI) or an anginal attack, all of the following are true statements EXCEPT

(A) anginal attacks usually last less than 10 to 15 minutes
(B) anginal attacks are often quickly relieved by rest, oxygen, or nitroglycerin
(C) only MI patients experience a shortness of breath, nausea, sweating, and weakness
(D) hypotension and shock are more commonly associated with MI patients

288. You are dispatched to a 62-year-old male with chest pain and difficulty breathing. As you open the door to the apartment, you find the patient pale and breathing 40 times a minute. After you begin to administer oxygen through a non-rebreather face mask, electrocardiogram (ECG) monitor, and IV line, you proceed to obtain a brief focused history. The patient has been a two-pack-a-day smoker for 40 years, hypertensive, who has been having 3 hours of the same epigastric pain that occurred with his first heart attack 5 years ago. As you continue to evaluate this chest pain patient, you begin to think about possible complications of an acute MI. All of the following are complications EXCEPT

(A) cardiogenic shock
(B) cardiac arrest
(C) congestive heart failure
(D) pneumonia

289. All of the following are signs of cardiogenic shock EXCEPT

(A) a rapid respiratory rate
(B) hot, red, flushed skin
(C) a rapid pulse
(D) a reduced level of consciousness

290. While cardiogenic shock frequently is caused by an acute MI, all of the following are additional causes of cardiogenic shock EXCEPT

(A) acute gastrointestinal (GI) bleeding
(B) progressive worsening of congestive heart failure caused by cardiomyopathy (heart muscle disease)
(C) worsening valvular heart disease
(D) rupture of papillary heart muscles or the interventricular septum

291. All of the following are symptoms or signs of congestive heart failure EXCEPT

(A) shortness of breath
(B) distended neck veins
(C) leg edema
(D) melena

292. All of the following are signs or symptoms of left-sided (left ventricular) CHF EXCEPT

(A) shortness of breath
(B) orthopnea (shortness of breath while lying down)
(C) pink frothy sputum
(D) abdominal swelling (ascites)

293. All of the following are signs or symptoms of right-sided (right ventricular) CHF EXCEPT

(A) abdominal swelling (ascites)
(B) distended neck veins
(C) bilateral leg edema
(D) moist rales on auscultation of the lungs

294. All of the following are symptoms or signs of a dissecting thoracic aortic aneurysm EXCEPT

  (A) bilateral leg edema
  (B) tearing anterior chest pain which may move down and to the back
  (C) asymmetric arterial pulses
  (D) signs of an acute cerebrovascular accident (stroke)

295. You are dispatched to a 70-year-old woman with a history of hypertension who is complaining of abdominal and back pain associated with nausea and vomiting. As you begin to examine the patient, you notice that her systolic blood pressure is 50 palpable and that she is cool, clammy, and lethargic. On abdominal examination, you find a markedly distended and tender abdomen with weak femoral pulses. This presentation is most consistent with the patient having

  (A) a kidney stone
  (B) a leaking abdominal aortic aneurysm
  (C) a ruptured abdominal aortic aneurysm
  (D) an intestinal virus

296. You are dispatched to the home of a 76-year-old woman who suddenly passed out. As you enter the patient's bedroom, you find her lying in bed, breathing 35 times per minute and appearing short of breath. The patient's husband states that she had been in bed for the past 5 days after returning home from the hospital. Evidently, the patient had slipped 2 weeks earlier, fractured her hip, and required surgical repair. The patient is able to tell you that she felt sudden right-sided pleuritic chest pain with severe difficulty breathing which began 1 hour ago. As you begin to examine the patient, you note that she has a red, hot, and swollen left calf and thigh. As you begin to take the patient's vital signs, she coughs up some blood. This patient's symptoms and signs are most likely due to

  (A) an acute cerebrovascular accident
  (B) an acute asthmatic attack
  (C) an acute pulmonary embolism
  (D) pneumonia

297. All of the following are risk factors for acute pulmonary embolism EXCEPT

  (A) a long bone fracture
  (B) taking birth control pills
  (C) a sedentary life-style
  (D) an acute sunburn

298. All of the following are causes of a hypertensive crisis EXCEPT

   (A) head trauma
   (B) a long bone fracture
   (C) pregnancy eclampsia or toxemia
   (D) acute pulmonary edema (left-sided heart failure)

299. All of the following are symptoms of a patient with a hypertensive crisis EXCEPT

   (A) diarrhea
   (B) headache
   (C) decreased level of consciousness
   (D) nosebleeds

300. You arrive to examine an 81-year-old "sick" man. The patient's neighbor states that he heard a loud sound from the hallway. As the neighbor went out to look, he found the patient unconscious. After 2 to 3 minutes the patient awakened. The patient admitted to feeling nauseous with abdominal cramps and was straining to move his bowels and felt dizzy and weak. Upon walking out in the hall to get help, he lost consciousness. The most likely cause of syncope in this patient is

   (A) an acute cardiovascular accident (CVA)
   (B) an acute duodenal ulcer
   (C) pneumonia
   (D) a vasovagal episode

301. All of the following are important to assess in a patient who has just had a syncopal episode EXCEPT

   (A) vital signs
   (B) the amount of time the patient was unconscious
   (C) if in the second or third trimester of pregnancy, the position the patient was in at the time of loss of consciousness
   (D) the patient's blood type

302. All of the following are true statements about a patient with syncope resulting from cardiac arrhythmias EXCEPT

   (A) the patient's heart rhythm before, during, and after the syncopal attack is normal sinus rhythm
   (B) the patient's heart rate shows severe bradycardia
   (C) the patient's heart rate shows severe tachycardia
   (D) the patient's heart rhythm shows a third-degree heart block

303. In a normal heart, electrical impulses are transmitted by way of the cardiac conduction system. Which of the following is the correct sequence for conducting the electrical message?

  (A) Sinus node, interatrial fibers, atrioventricular (AV) node, right and left bundle branches, bundle of His, Purkinje fibers, ventricular myocardium

  (B) AV node, interatrial fibers, sino-atrial (SA) node, bundle of His, Purkinje fibers, ventricular myocardium, right and left bundle branches

  (C) sinus node, interatrial fibers, bundle of His, AV node, right and left bundle branches, Purkinje fibers, ventricular myocardium

  (D) SA node, interatrial fibers, AV node, bundle of His, right and left bundle branches, Purkinje fibers, ventricular myocardium

304. The most commonly identified initial rhythm at the time of cardiac arrest is

  (A) asystole
  (B) ventricular tachycardia
  (C) ventricular fibrillation
  (D) normal sinus rhythm

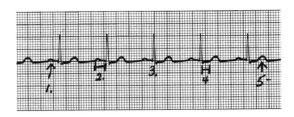

305. Based on the five items labeled in the above ECG strip, complete this matching column:

  (A) The QRS complex represents ventricular depolarization, resulting in ventricular contraction

  (B) The ST segment represents the beginning of ventricular depolarization

  (C) The P wave represents atrial depolarization, resulting in atrial contraction

  (D) The PR interval is an electrical impulse passing through the AV node

  (E) The T wave represents the completion of ventricular depolarization

  1. _____
  2. _____
  3. _____
  4. _____
  5. _____

306. For the following cardiac rhythms, correctly match the names:
(A) Normal sinus rhythm
(B) Ventricular tachycardia
(C) Sinus bradycardia
(D) Asystole
(E) Ventricular fibrillation
(F) Sinus tachycardia
(G) Premature ventricular contractions
1. ——— 5. ———
2. ——— 6. ———
3. ——— 7. ———
4. ———

1.

2.

3.

4.

5.

6.

7.

307. Defibrillation is defined as the application of an electric shock to the heart to restore an effective heart rhythm. Defibrillation should be applied in which of the following dysrhythmias?

(A) Ventricular fibrillation and brady-arrhythmia
(B) Ventricular tachycardia with a pulse
(C) Ventricular fibrillation and ventricular tachycardia with a pulse
(D) Ventricular fibrillation and ventricular tachycardia without a pulse

308. You are dispatched to a 70-year-old male with "possible cardiac arrest." As you approach the man's home, you find the patient lying on the floor in cardiac arrest, pulseless and apneic. Your first action should be to

(A) begin an intravenous line for access
(B) perform endotracheal intubation
(C) take a quick look with an automated external defibrillator (AED) and, if indicated, defibrillate
(D) begin cardiopulmonary resuscitation (CPR)

309. All of the following are indications for use of an AED EXCEPT

(A) patient must be in cardiac arrest
(B) patient with chest pain
(C) cardiac arrest patient in ventricular tachycardia
(D) cardiac arrest patient in ventricular fibrillation

310. While driving to get gas, you are "flagged down" by a person who is screaming that someone just collapsed in the hardware store. As you kneel to assess the patient, it is clear that an approximately 60-year-old man is not responsive, apneic, and pulseless. As you begin to apply an AED, the correct sequence to follow is

(A) turn on the power, attach the defibrillation pads to the cable and then to the patient's chest, stop CPR, press the analyze button, if advised to shock, clear everyone from contact with the patient, press to deliver the shock

(B) stop CPR, turn on the power, attach the defibrillation pads to the cable and then to the patient's chest, press the analyze button, if advised to shock, shock immediately

(C) attach the defibrillation pads to the patient's chest and then to the cable, turn on the power, press the analyze button, clear everyone from contact with the patient, press to deliver the shock

(D) turn on the power, stop CPR, press the analyze button, if advised to shock, shock immediately

311. In providing emergency care for a cardiac arrest victim, after setting up the AED, you press the analyze button. Which of the following is a correct statement concerning this analysis period?

(A) Most AEDs require 5 to 15 seconds to analyze the rhythm, and you must not touch or move the patient during that period

(B) Most AEDs require 30 seconds to analyze the rhythm, and you must not touch or move the patient during that period

(C) Most AEDs analyze the rhythm immediately, and you can continue CPR during that period

(D) Most AEDs require 15 to 30 seconds to analyze the rhythm, and you can continue CPR during that period

312. Both automatic and semiautomatic defibrillators will analyze a cardiac arrest patient's heart rhythm and determine whether a shock is indicated. However, the most important difference between these two types of defibrillators is that

(A) the automatic is half the weight of the semiautomatic
(B) the automatic can shock only at 200 J while the semiautomatic can go up to 360 J
(C) the automatic, after warning the operator, will automatically deliver a shock; the semi-automatic will advise the operator to shock, but the operator must push the button to do so
(D) the automatic will advise you to administer particular IV medications for nonshockable rhythms, while the semiautomatic does not have this capability

313. In using an AED for a cardiac arrest patient, after delivering the third shock, the EMT-I should proceed to

(A) immediately transport the patient to the hospital
(B) do CPR for 1 minute and then check for a pulse; if the patient is pulseless, provide advanced life support according to the local protocol
(C) check for a pulse; if it is present, push the analyze button of the AED and shock if advised to do so
(D) do CPR for 5 minutes, press the analyze button, and shock if advised to do so

314. In using an AED, if at any time the patient develops a pulse, one should proceed to

(A) disconnect the AED and monitor the patient's vital signs every 5 minutes
(B) press the analyze button and shock if advised to do so
(C) start CPR for 1 minute, press the analyze button, and shock if advised to do so
(D) monitor the patient, administer further care according to the local protocol, and transport the patient to the hospital

315. All of the following are contraindications to the use of an AED EXCEPT

(A) a 110-lb 15-year-old girl in cardiac arrest
(B) a 60-lb 6-year-old boy in cardiac arrest
(C) a 70-lb 92-year-old female in cardiac arrest
(D) a 56-year-old male, unconscious, with a strong pulse

316. You are dispatched to an "unconscious" victim and upon your arrival find a 75-year-old male who is pulseless and apneic. Since you are equipped with a manual defibrillator, you should proceed to do all of the following EXCEPT

(A) bare the patient's chest and apply the gel pad electrodes or apply gel to the paddles

(B) set the energy level to 360 J and charge the defibrillator

(C) apply the paddles to the proper locations and reverify the dysrhythmia

(D) announce to "clear" from the patient, verify that everyone is clear from patient contact, and press both paddles' buttons to deliver the shock

317. You are in the middle of attempting to resuscitate a 57-year-old female cardiac arrest victim. After completing a series of three stacked shocks, you perform CPR for 1 minute and check for a pulse. Since the patient is still pulseless, you begin to deliver advanced cardiac life support according to the local protocol. After the patient is intubated and IV access is established, you consider the administration of cardiac drugs. Epinephrine is indicated in all of the following dysrhythmias EXCEPT

(A) ventricular fibrillation

(B) asystole

(C) frequent premature ventricular contractions (PVCs)

(D) pulseless electrical activity (PEA)

318. Which of the following are accepted as indications for the use of IV atropine in acute cardiac care?

(A) Asystole and ventricular fibrillation

(B) Ventricular tachycardia with a pulse and atrial fibrillation

(C) Atrial flutter and ventricular fibrillation

(D) Asystole and hemodynamically significant bradycardias

319. All of the following are indications for the use of lidocaine in acute cardiac care EXCEPT

(A) ventricular fibrillation

(B) ventricular tachycardia without a pulse

(C) ventricular tachycardia with a pulse

(D) idioventricular rhythm

CARDIAC EMERGENCIES

282. The answer is C. (Mosby, *Cardiac Emergencies.*) Hypertension, cigarette smoking, diabetes, a family history of heart attack or sudden death, male sex, an elevated cholesterol level, obesity, a sedentary life-style, and stress are all risk factors for cardiac disease. Insomnia is not related to cardiac risk factors.

283. The answer is B. (Mosby, *Cardiac Emergencies.*) (A), (C), and (D) are all correct. (B) is incorrect because EMT-Is must have medical control authorization to assist a patient in administering nitroglycerin tablets or spray.

284. The answer is A. (Mosby, *Cardiac Emergencies.*) Headache, tingling under the tongue, hypotension, dizziness, flushing, tachycardia, nausea, and a rash are common side effects of sublingual nitroglycerin. An oral fungal infection is not related to sublingual nitroglycerin tablet and spray administration.

285. The answer is C. (Mosby, *Cardiac Emergencies.*) (A), (B), and (D) are correct steps in helping a patient administer prescribed nitroglycerin. (C) is incorrect because you should not shake nitroglycerin spray before its administration. Shaking results in administering an incorrect dose.

286. The answer is A. (Mosby, *Cardiac Emergencies.*) (B), (C), and (D) are contraindications to the administration of nitroglycerin. If the patient took three doses of nitroglycerin just before the EMT-I's arrival, additional nitroglycerin is usually contraindicated. However, the EMT-I should follow local medical control protocol on this issue.

287. The answer is C. (Mosby, *Cardiac Emergencies.*) (A), (B), and (D) are correct. (C) is incorrect because both angina and myocardial infarction patients may complain of shortness of breath, nausea, sweating, and weakness.

288. The answer is D. (Mosby, *Cardiac Emergencies.*) Cardiogenic shock, cardiac arrest, congestive heart failure, syncope, cardiac arrhythmias, and cardiac rupture are all complications of an acute MI. Pneumonia is not a complication of an acute MI.

289. The answer is B. (Brady, *Fluids and Shock.*) (A), (C), (D), hypotension, cool clammy skin, decreased oxygen saturation on pulse oximetry, and decreased urine output are all signs of cardiogenic shock. (B) is not such a sign.

290. The answer is A. (Brady, *Fluids and Shock.*) (B), (C), and (D) are additional causes of cardiogenic shock. Acute GI bleeding may cause hypovolemic shock from blood loss but not cardiogenic shock.

291. The answer is D. (Mosby, *Cardiac Emergencies.*) Shortness of breath, distended neck veins, leg edema, pink frothy sputum, moist rales and wheezes on auscultation, abdominal swelling, tachycardia, sleeping on an increasing number of pillows at night, and awakening from sleep short of breath are some of the symptoms or signs of congestive heart failure. Melena is defined as black tarry stools, which is a symptom of upper GI bleeding. It is not a symptom or sign of CHF.

292. The answer is D. (Mosby, *Cardiac Emergencies.*) Shortness of breath, orthopnea, pink frothy sputum, and moist rales and wheezes on auscultation are signs and symptoms of left-sided CHF. Abdominal swelling is a sign of right-sided CHF.

293. The answer is D. (Mosby, *Cardiac Emergencies.*) Abdominal swelling, distended neck veins, bilateral leg edema, and swelling of the liver and spleen are signs or symptoms of right-sided CHF. Moist rales on auscultation of the lungs are a sign of left-sided CHF.

294. The answer is A. (Mosby, *Cardiac Emergencies.*) (B), (C), (D), MI, pericardial tamponade, and syncope are all symptoms or signs of a dissecting thoracic aortic aneurysm. Bilateral leg edema is not.

295. The answer is C. (Mosby, *Cardiac Emergencies.*) A patient with a leaking or ruptured abdominal aortic aneurysm frequently complains of back pain, abdominal pain, nausea, vomiting, and signs of shock. A palpable abdominal mass may be present with a leaking abdominal aortic aneurysm. However, a ruptured abdominal aortic aneurysm usually is not palpable and produces a very distended and tender abdomen. A kidney stone usually produces unilateral back or side pain without signs of shock with normal femoral pulses. An intestinal virus may produce abdominal pain, nausea and vomiting, and abdominal distention, but usually without signs of shock and with normal femoral pulses.

296. The answer is C. (Mosby, *Cardiac Emergencies.*) Some of the symptoms and signs of acute pulmonary embolism are syncope, acute onset of pleuritic increases on taking a deep breath, chest pain, shortness of breath, respiratory distress, coughing up blood, wheezing, hypotension, and cardiac arrest.

297. The answer is D. (Mosby, *Cardiac Emergencies.*) A long bone fracture, birth control pills, a sedentary life-style, obesity, thrombophlebitis, pregnancy, blood disorders, and a patient lying on an operating table for several hours are risk factors for acute pulmonary embolism. An acute sunburn is not a risk factor.

298. The answer is B. (Mosby, *Cardiac Emergencies.*) Head trauma, pregnancy eclampsia or toxemia, acute pulmonary edema, certain drug ingestions (e.g., amphetamines, cocaine, thyroid hormone), acute kidney infection or disease, a dissecting thoracic aortic aneurysm, and acute intracerebral strokes and hemorrhages are all causes of a hypertensive crisis. A long bone fracture is not related to a hypertensive crisis.

299. The answer is A. (Mosby, *Cardiac Emergencies.*) Headache, a decreased level of consciousness, nosebleeds, acute visual problems, nausea and vomiting, chest pain, shortness of breath, and dizziness may all be symptoms of a hypertensive crisis.

300. The answer is D. (Mosby, *Cardiac Emergencies.*) A vasovagal episode, cardiac arrhythmias, central nervous system disorders (seizures, strokes/transient ischemic attacks, intracerebral hemorrhage), hyperventilation, anxiety, over- or underactive thyroid disease, hypoglycemia, a drug or medication overdose, the Valsalva maneuver, and intravascular hypovolemia may all cause syncope.

301. The answer is D. (Mosby, *Cardiac Emergencies.*) (D) is not significant. (A), (B), (C), symptoms and signs of orthostasis (decrease in blood pressure going from lying to sitting or from sitting to standing with an increase in the pulse rate), any whiteness and signs of a seizure are all important parts of the assessment of a patient with syncope.

302. The answer is A. (Brady, *Appendix I Defibrillation.*) If the heart rhythm before, during, and after a syncopal episode is normal sinus rhythm, a cardiac arrhythmia cannot be the cause of the syncope. One must search for another cause.

303. The answer is D. (Brady, *Appendix I Defibrillation.*) (D) is the correct sequence of the cardiac conduction system in a normal heart.

304. The answer is C. (Brady, *Appendix I Defibrillation.*) Ventricular fibrillation is the most commonly identified initial rhythm in cardiac arrest patients. Asystole and ventricular tachycardia are also seen in cardiac arrest patients, but not a normal sinus rhythm.

305. Answers.
1.   C
2.   D
3.   A
4.   B
5.   E

306 **Answers**
1. F
2. G
3. A
4. E
5. D
6. C
7. B

307. **The answer is D.** (Mosby, *Cardiac Emergencies.*) Defibrillation should be applied immediately to a cardiac arrest patient in ventricular fibrillation or in ventricular tachycardia without a pulse. A patient in ventricular tachycardia with a pulse usually is treated initially with intravenous medications such as lidocaine. Cardiac arrest patients with bradyarrhythmias are never defibrillated. They are treated with intravenous medications such as epinephrine and atropine.

308. **The answer is C.** (Mosby, *Cardiac Emergencies.*) Early defibrillation is the first priority in the care of a cardiac arrest patient. If indicated, providing an electrical shock may restore an effective heart rhythm immediately. If a second EMT-I is present, he or she should begin CPR.

309. **The answer is B.** (Mosby, *Cardiac Emergencies.*) (A), (C), and (D) are the indications for the use of an AED. It is essential to document that the patient is truly in cardiac arrest. There is no role for an AED in chest pain patients.

310. **The answer is A.** (Mosby, *Cardiac Emergencies.* Brady, *Appendix I Defibrillation.*) (A) is the correct sequence to use in applying an AED.

311. **The answer is A.** (Mosby, *Cardiac Emergencies.*) With any patient movement, the AED may incorrectly interpret a stable rhythm as a shockable rhythm. If, while you are transporting a patient, he or she goes into cardiac arrest, before pressing the AEDs analyze button you must stop the ambulance and turn off the motor.

312. **The answer is C.** (Mosby, *Cardiac Emergencies.*) (C) is the most important difference between these two defibrillators. (A) is incorrect because there is no difference in size or weight between these two defibrillators. Both defibrillators are capable of shocking between 200 and 360 J. Neither defibrillator will advise you to administer any medications to a patient.

313. **The answer is B.** (Mosby, *Cardiac Emergencies.*) (B) is the correct approach to emergently treating a cardiac arrest patient after delivering the third shock of three stacked shocks. (A) is incorrect because the EMT-I has been trained to continue properly treating the patient, according to (B). (C) is incorrect because one never pushes the button to analyze the rhythm if the patient has a pulse. (D) is incorrect because one should do CPR for only 1 minute and then proceed according to (B).

314. The answer is D. (Mosby, *Cardiac Emergencies.*) (D) is the correct approach to a cardiac arrest patient who develops a pulse. (A) is incorrect because one should never disconnect the AED from a cardiac arrest patient until arrival at the emergency department. The AED provides a means of monitoring the heart rhythm as well as being immediately available if the patient goes back into cardiac arrest. (B) and (C) are incorrect because in a patient with a pulse, one should never analyze the heart rhythm with an AED and never start CPR.

315. The answer is A. (Mosby, *Cardiac Emergencies.*) (A) is correct because most authorities recommend that AEDs should not be used on anyone under 12 years old or weighing less than 90 lb (child or adult). (B) and (C) are incorrect because these patients do not fit the previously mentioned guidelines. (D) is incorrect because the patient has a pulse and is not in cardiac arrest and thus is not a candidate for the AED.

316. The answer is B. (Mosby, *Cardiac Emergencies.*) (B) is incorrect because the first energy level setting is 200 J. (A), (C), and (D) are parts of the process of applying a manual defibrillator to a cardiac arrest patient.

317. The answer is C. (Mosby, *Cardiac Emergencies.*) Frequent PVCs are never treated with epinephrine. Ventricular fibrillation, asystole, PEA, and ventricular tachycardia without a pulse are all indications for treatment with intravenous epinephrine in a cardiac arrest patient.

318. The answer is D. (Mosby, *Cardiac Emergencies.*) In acute cardiac care, atropine is indicated in (D). While asystole is an indication for atropine, the rhythms in (A), (B), and (C) are not.

319. The answer is D. (Mosby, *Cardiac Emergencies.*) Ventricular fibrillation, ventricular tachycardia without a pulse, ventricular tachycardia with a pulse, and frequent PVCs are indications for the use of IV lidocaine. An idioventricular rhythm is not an indication. IV lidocaine use in a patient in idioventricular rhythm could result in asystole by eliminating this ventricular-originating rhythm.

MEDICAL
EMERGENCIES

In this chapter, you will review:

- signs of asthmatic attack

- strokes, seizures, and coma

- diabetic emergencies

MEDICAL EMERGENCIES

Directions: Each item below contains four suggested responses. Select the **one best** response to each item.

320. Which of the following sequences BEST describes the pathophysiology of anaphylactic shock?

   (A) Antigen (foreign substance), mast cell, histamine, antibody
   (B) Antibody, antigen (foreign substance), histamine, mast cell
   (C) Antigen (foreign substance), antibody, mast cell, histamine
   (D) Mast cell, histamine, antibody, antigen (foreign substance)

321. Which of the following are common signs and symptoms of anaphylactic shock?

   (A) Fever, earache, nausea, coughing up blood
   (B) Mouth-hand-tongue swelling, skin hives, stridor, wheezing
   (C) Seizure, fever, ankle pain, blotchy skin
   (D) Neck pain, nausea and vomiting, heart murmur, diarrhea

322. You are dispatched to a 20-year-old man who was stung by a bee and is complaining of difficulty breathing. He is wheezing with stridor and with a swollen tongue and lips and skin hives. After assessing this patient, you note that his blood pressure is 70/50 with a pulse of 120 per minute. All of the following may be part of the treatment of this patient EXCEPT

   (A) non-rebreather mask at 10 to 15 liters per minute or nasal oxygen at 5 to 6 liters per minute
   (B) intravenous (IV) saline or lactated Ringer's solution wide open
   (C) Lasix 20–40-mg IV bolus
   (D) epinephrine 0.1–0.5-mg sub-cutaneous injection

323. All of the following are components of the pathophysiology of asthma EXCEPT

(A) fever and sore throat
(B) bronchospasm
(C) increased mucus production
(D) airway swelling and edema

324. All of the following are known to trigger asthmatic attacks EXCEPT

(A) respiratory infections and irritants
(B) exercise and emotions
(C) chemicals and street drugs
(D) antibiotics and a Proventil inhaler

325. The following are signs or symptoms of an asthmatic attack EXCEPT

(A) hemoptysis (coughing up blood)
(B) shortness of breath
(C) coughing with or without sputum
(D) tachypnea, anxiety, and agitation

326. You are sent to an apartment to see a 23-year-old male asthmatic patient who is complaining of having difficulty breathing for the past 10 hours despite the frequent use of his Proventil inhaler. In performing a physical assessment of this patient, which of the following is a sign that the patient is having a serious asthmatic attack?

(A) Fever
(B) Loud wheezing
(C) A productive cough
(D) A silent chest

327. As you arrive to see a 26-year-old female patient with shortness of breath, you find that the patient had agreed to watch a friend's cat for the past 2 days. She states that after the first few hours of making contact with the cat, she has had itchy tearing eyes, a continuous cough, and now worsening wheezing with shortness of breath. All of the following may be part of the emergency care of a patient with an acute asthmatic attack EXCEPT

(A) calm and reassure the patient
(B) administer an aerosol bronchodilator such as albuterol (Proventil), metaproterenol (Alupent), or isoetharine (Bronkosol)
(C) administer IV epinephrine 1.0 mg of 1:10,000 solution
(D) administer high-concentration oxygen 10 to 15 liters per minute by non-rebreather mask

328. All of the following are true statements about status asthmaticus EXCEPT

(A) it is defined as a severe prolonged asthmatic attack which does not respond to standard medications
(B) it requires immediate transport
(C) prehospital emergency care is the same as that for treating an acute asthmatic attack, including the possible need for urgent endotracheal intubation
(D) it often requires giving three to four times the standard dose of epinephrine

329. All of the following medical conditions may cause hyperventilation EXCEPT

   (A) acute pulmonary embolism
   (B) acute myocardial infarction
   (C) central nervous system (CNS) lesions, strokes, infections, head trauma
   (D) a narcotic overdose

330. All of the following are priorities in the treatment of a patient with chronic obstructive pulmonary disease (COPD) EXCEPT

   (A) transport the patient in the semi-sitting position
   (B) administer IV normal saline at 300 mL per hour
   (C) administer a bronchodilator
   (D) administer oxygen

331. You arrive at the apartment of a 54-year-old man who is complaining of "difficulty breathing." Upon further questioning, the patient complains of a numb and tingling feeling in his fingers and toes and around his mouth and is dizzy. Your assessment reveals that the patient's respiratory rate is 40 per minute, blood pressure is 110/70, and pulse is 110 per minute. Which of the following is the correct approach to treating hyperventilation?

   (A) Make the patient rebreathe in a paper bag
   (B) Plug the portals in an oxygen mask so that the patient can rebreathe in the mask
   (C) Assume that there is a medical problem causing the patient to hyperventilate and administer oxygen at 3 to 4 liters per minute. If pulse oximetry shows hypoxia, increase to 15 liters per minute
   (D) Assume that the patient always has anxiety hyperventilation and advise him to relax

332. All of the following are at risk for developing pulmonary emboli EXCEPT

   (A) patients with thrombophlebitis (vein inflammation)
   (B) patients on prolonged bed rest
   (C) patients undergoing surgery for several hours
   (D) patients with minor hand injuries

333. All of the following are signs or symptoms of pulmonary embolism EXCEPT

(A) melena (black stools)
(B) acute onset of pleuritic chest pain
(C) syncope
(D) hemoptysis (coughing up blood)

334. Which of the following BEST describes the mechanism of a spontaneous pneumothorax?

(A) Acute collapse of a lung caused by a penetrating injury
(B) Acute collapse of a lung caused by a gunshot wound
(C) Acute accumulation of air in the pleural space
(D) Acute collapse of a lung caused by a needle biopsy of the lung

335. All of the following are signs of a tension pneumothorax EXCEPT

(A) acute respiratory distress
(B) decreased or absent breath sounds on the involved side
(C) focal leg weakness
(D) trachea deviated away from the involved side

336. All of the following are signs or symptoms of a stroke EXCEPT

(A) paralysis
(B) slurred speech
(C) altered level of consciousness
(D) frequent urination

337. You are dispatched to a skilled nursing facility because of a change in one of the elderly residents. Upon arrival, you find a 72-year-old female who appears lethargic, is unable to speak, and has paralysis of the right arm and leg. All of the following demonstrate the importance of airway management in a patient with a stroke EXCEPT

(A) laryngitis is a common complication of a stroke
(B) if an acute stroke patient is unable to protect his or her airway, he or she may aspirate oral secretions and/or vomitus into the lungs
(C) one should consider endotracheal intubation if the patient is unable to manage his or her airway
(D) one should not allow a stroke victim to take anything by mouth because of the uncertainty of airway protection

338. All of the following are intracranial causes of coma EXCEPT

(A) stroke
(B) brain tumor
(C) narcotic overdose
(D) intracranial hemorrhage

339. All of the following are causes of coma which originate outside the nervous system EXCEPT

(A) alcohol and drug overdose
(B) kidney failure
(C) ovarian failure
(D) metabolic abnormalities demonstrated in electrolyte abnormalities in the blood, such as high or low blood sugar

340. Fill in the blanks for the AEIOU–TIPS mnemonic for the causes of coma:

A   _____
E   _____
I   _____
O   _____
U   _____
T   _____
I   _____
P   _____
S   _____

341. You are dispatched to a 51-year-old unconscious female patient. Upon arrival at the patient's home, you find the patient lying on the floor, unresponsive to any verbal or painful stimuli. The patient's husband states that he just awoke and found her lying there. All of the following are priorities in providing emergency care to a comatose patient EXCEPT

- (A) administer a small glass of orange juice with added sugar by mouth
- (B) establish and maintain an airway and consider the need for endotracheal intubation
- (C) following the local protocol, obtain fingerstick glucose and, if it is less than 60, administer 1 ampule (25 g) of $D_{50}W$
- (D) if there is no response to $D_{50}W$, follow the local protocol and administer IV naloxone (Narcan)

342. All of the following are different types of seizures EXCEPT

- (A) generalized motor seizure (grand mal)
- (B) focal motor seizure
- (C) anxiety seizure
- (D) behavioral seizure

343. You arrive at an office building and find a 51-year-old female surrounded by her coworkers. Evidently, the patient began to have facial and muscle twitching and then fell to the floor and was described as having generalized tonic-clonic muscle contractions for about 8 to 10 minutes before they stopped. As you kneel to assess the patient, she begins to have another grand mal seizure. All of the following are important parts of the prehospital emergency care of a seizure patient EXCEPT

- (A) maintain an open airway
- (B) prepare to provide suctioning of oral secretions and/or vomitus during and after the seizure
- (C) actively restrain the patient to a long spine board to limit the muscle contractions
- (D) administer high-concentration O_2 and an ECG monitor and establish an IV line

344. All of the following are serious causes of headache EXCEPT

- (A) intracranial bleeding
- (B) meningitis or encephalitis
- (C) anxiety
- (D) brain tumor

345. You are dispatched to a nursing home because an 80-year-old man has been complaining of stomach pain. The pain is located in the left lower abdomen and has increased in intensity over the past 2 hours. All of the following are parts of the emergency care rendered to a patient with abdominal pain EXCEPT

    (A) airway, oxygen, and assisted ventilation if needed
    ·(B) allow clear liquids by mouth
    (C) be prepared to suction the mouth if the patient vomits
    (D) administer 500 to 1000 mL IV normal saline or lactated Ringer's if the patient is hypotensive or dehydrated

346. All of the following are causes of upper GI bleeding EXCEPT

    (A) peptic ulcer disease
    ·(B) hemorrhoids
    (C) esophageal varices
    (D) acute gastritis

347. All of the following are causes of lower GI bleeding EXCEPT

    ·(A) appendicitis
    (B) colon cancer
    (C) hemorrhoids
    (D) diverticulosis

348. All of the following are signs or symptoms of hypoglycemia EXCEPT

    (A) palpitations
    ·(B) fever
    (C) sweating
    (D) altered level of consciousness

349. While treating a minor injury at an amusement park, you are asked to evaluate an unconscious 26-year-old woman. As you kneel to assess the patient, you are told that she is an insulin-dependent diabetic. Her friend informs you that she took insulin this morning but did not eat breakfast or lunch. All of the following are priorities in providing emergency care to a hypoglycemic patient EXCEPT

    (A) assess the airway and assist respirations as needed
    (B) administer oxygen at 6 liters per minute
    (C) if the patient is responsive, give sugar dissolved in orange juice
    ·(D) administer SQ epinephrine 0.3 mL of 1:1,000 solution

350. All of the following are signs or symptoms of diabetic ketoacidosis EXCEPT

    ,(A) high blood pressure
    ·(B) fruity breath odor
    (C) increased thirst, hunger, and urination
    (D) altered mental status

351. You are dispatched to a skilled nursing facility to see a 70-year-old man with a history of diabetes who is much less responsive than usual. All of the following are signs of hyperosmolar hyperglycemic nonketotic coma in this patient EXCEPT

    '(A) fruity breath odor
    (B) dehydration
    (C) gradual deterioration over 4 to 5 days
    (D) altered mental status, even unresponsiveness

352. You arrive at the home of a 23-year-old male "sick diabetic" and find the patient in bed, lethargic and hot to the touch. His mother states that he has had the flu for the past 2 days with fever, chills, abdominal cramps, and diarrhea. Because his appetite has been poor, he has not taken insulin for 2 days. All of the following are parts of the emergent care given to a diabetic by an EMT-Intermediate (EMT-I) EXCEPT

(A) maintain the airway, administer oxygen, assist ventilation, including endotracheal intubation if necessary

(B) administer the patient's standard daily dose of insulin SQ

(C) monitor vital signs and ECG

(D) per the local protocol, administer $D_{50}W$

353. All of the following are routes of exposure to poison EXCEPT

(A) evaporation

(B) ingestion

(C) absorption

(D) injection

354. You are dispatched to the home of a 20-year-old boy who drank a few glasses of an unknown poison. Upon arrival you find a lethargic male lying on the garage floor. All of the following are important pieces of information to obtain from a poisoned patient EXCEPT

(A) amount of poison ingested

(B) time of ingestion

(C) ingested substance hot or cold

(D) name of substance ingested

355. As your partner obtains a history from a poisoned patient, you begin to perform a physical assessment. All of the following are important areas to assess in a poisoned patient EXCEPT

(A) temperature

(B) pulse

(C) blood pressure

(D) presence of swollen glands

356. You arrive at the home of an 11-year-old girl who admits taking 30 Tylenol tablets 25 minutes ago. An empty bottle of 500-mg extra-strength Tylenol tablets is found on the floor. After assessing the child and instituting emergency care for a poisoned patient, you consider administering syrup of ipecac to induce vomiting. All of the following are aspects of the correct use of syrup of ipecac EXCEPT

(A) confirm the written or verbal local protocol from medical direction

(B) patient is unresponsive

(C) adult dose is 30 mL and child dose is 15 mL

(D) after receiving syrup of ipecac, the patient needs to drink several glasses of water

357. You arrive at the scene of a fire and find an unconscious 62-year-old female being carried out of a burning building. The fire fighters state that she was unconscious on a bed in a smoke-filled room. Which of the following is the BEST sign that this patient may be suffering from carbon monoxide poisoning?

(A) The patient has a rapid pulse and high blood pressure

(B) The pulse oximetry reading shows a very low level of oxygen-saturated hemoglobin

(C) The patient's breath has a sweet, fruity odor

(D) The patient is a victim of a fire

358. You arrive at an outdoor basketball court on a 95° day and find a 17-year-old boy complaining of severe muscle cramps in the abdomen and legs. Evidently, he has played full-court basketball for over 2 hours without a break. All of the following are parts of the emergency care given to a patient suffering from heat cramps EXCEPT

(A) initially, while assessing the patient, do not move the patient from the basketball court

(B) administer 500-1000 mL of normal saline

(C) do not give salt pills

(D) if the patient is alert, allow him or her to take sips of cool water

359. You are working as an EMT-I for a beach club and are asked to evaluate a 14-year-old girl who has "had too much sun." The patient complains of being thirsty and tired and of having a headache. Your assessment finds her pale, diaphoretic, warm to touch, and hypotensive. The emergency care of a patient with heat exhaustion is the same as that of a heat cramps patient EXCEPT

(A) remove to a cool environment

(B) administer high-concentration oxygen by non-rebreather mask (15-liters-per-minute flow rate)

(C) start an IV and fluid bolus according to the local protocol

(D) give the patient sips of cool water

360. As you finish providing care to the patient in question 359, you are pulled away by a frantic teenager to see a 17-year-old boy found in the dunes of the beach. This young man is speaking incoherently and becomes unresponsive in your presence. Upon further assessment, he has very hot, dry skin and has only a palpable blood pressure of 50. In providing emergency care to this patient with heat stroke, which of the following is the most important?

(A) ECG monitor

(B) Rapid cooling

(C) High-concentration oxygen

(D) Transport to the hospital

361. You are assigned to a homeless man found on a freezing cold night in a back alley. This 64-year-old male is lying on the ground without any shoes or socks. The patient's toes appear waxy bluish-white, hard, cold, and not sensitive to pain. Emergency care for a patient with frostbite includes all of the following EXCEPT

(A) do not break any blisters
(B) do not allow the patient to smoke or drink alcohol
(C) do not rewarm the frostbite injury in the field
(D) do not treat the patient for hypothermia until the frostbite area has been treated

362. You are dispatched to an elderly man found in the snow. You find an 80-year-old male who is unresponsive, pulseless, and apneic. There are no witnesses to how long the patient has been on the ground. In administering emergency care to this hypothermic patient, all of the following are true EXCEPT

(A) begin cardiopulmonary resuscitation (CPR) but check a pulse for 2 minutes before beginning chest compressions
(B) administer IV (ideally, warmed) normal saline or lactated Ringer's solution 500–1000 mL as quickly as possible, per the local protocol
(C) remove wet clothing and keep the patient in a warm environment
(D) follow the local protocol on rewarming, at least by covering the patient with blankets in a warm ambulance; if transport time is more than 1 hour, consider placing hot packs over the carotids, head, lateral thorax, and groin

MEDICAL EMERGENCIES

320. **The answer is C.** (Mosby, *Medical Emergencies.*) The pathophysiology of anaphylactic shock follows the sequence of an antigen (foreign substance), which triggers the production of an antibody. The antigen-antibody complex causes circulating mast cells to release chemical substances such as histamine, and this produces an anaphylactic reaction.

321. **The answer is B.** (Mosby, *Medical Emergencies.*) In addition to (B), tingling, itching or burning skin, hypotension (low blood pressure), tachycardia, sweating, a decrease in mental status, a weak or thready pulse, accessory muscle use, cyanosis, and anxiety are all signs and symptoms of anaphylactic shock.

322. **The answer is C.** (Mosby, *Medical Emergencies.*) (A), (B), and (D) are all parts of the emergency treatment of anaphylactic shock, along with IV Benadryl and nebulized bronchodilator with albuterol (Proventil, Ventolin) or isoetharine (Bronkosol). Place the patient in a position of comfort and attempt to remove the "stinger" (venom sac) with a flat object. IV Lasix has no place in the treatment of an anaphylactic shock or reaction.

323. **The answer is A.** (Mosby, *Medical Emergencies.*) Bronchospasm, increased mucus production, and swelling and edema as well as increased inflammatory cell proliferation are all parts of the pathophysiology of asthma. While fever and a sore throat may aggravate asthma, they are not part of its pathophysiology.

324. **The answer is D.** (Mosby, *Medical Emergencies.*) (A), (B), (C), allergens, and changes in environmental conditions are all known to trigger asthmatic attacks. Antibiotics and a Proventil inhaler are not known to trigger asthmatic attacks. A Proventil inhaler frequently is used to treat an asthmatic attack.

325. The answer is A. (Mosby, *Medical Emergencies.*) (B), (C), (D), audible wheezes, difficulty moving air in and out, mild cyanosis, tachycardia, hypertension, and decreased oxygen saturation on pulse oximetry are all signs or symptoms of an asthmatic attack. Hemoptysis (coughing up blood) is not.

326. The answer is D. (Mosby, *Medical Emergencies.*) A silent chest refers to the absence of breath sounds on auscultation and documents that the airways are very narrowed. It is a sign that an asthmatic patient is seriously ill. Other signs of a serious asthmatic attack are altered level of consciousness, cyanosis, marked diaphoresis, and a patient stating that he or she is too tired to breathe. Fever, loud wheezing, and a productive cough may all be part of an asthma patient's presentation but are not individual signs of a serious attack.

327. The answer is C. (Mosby, *Medical Emergencies.*) (A), (B), (D), sitting upright, rapid transport, repeating vital signs, an IV line, an electrocardiogram (ECG) monitor, pulse oximetry, 0.25 mL subcutaneous (SQ) terbutaline (Brethine), SQ 0.1–0.5 mL epinephrine (Adrenalin), and endotracheal intubation are all possible parts of the emergency care of an asthmatic patient. (C) is incorrect because you do not give IV epinephrine to an asthmatic patient. You may need to give SQ epinephrine 0.1–0.5 mL to an asthmatic patient.

328. The answer is D. (Mosby, *Medical Emergencies.*) (A), (B), and (C) are correct. (D) is incorrect because one administers the standard dose of epinephrine (0.1–0.5 mL) only SQ.

329. The answer is D. (Mosby, *Medical Emergencies.*) (A), (B), and (C) are some of the causes of hyperventilation. Additional causes are congestive heart failure, fever, infections, hyperthyroidism (overactive), hypoxia, spontaneous pneumothorax, metabolic acidosis, certain drugs (epinephrine, cocaine, aspirin, amphetamines) and psychogenic factors. A narcotic overdose usually produces hypoventilation.

330. The answer is B. (Mosby, *Medical Emergencies.*) (A), (C), (D), and encouraging the patient to cough up secretions are priorities in the treatment of a COPD patient. (B) is incorrect because starting an IV line with normal saline to keep the vein open (KVO) is the correct treatment.

331. The answer is C. (Mosby, *Medical Emergencies.*) (A) and (B) are incorrect because rebreathing causes a significant decrease in the oxygen available for the patient, resulting in serious hypoxia. (D) is incorrect because hyperventilation may be caused by numerous serious medical problems.

332. The answer is D. (Mosby, *Medical Emergencies.*) Thrombophlebitis, prolonged bed rest, undergoing surgery for several hours, obesity, sedentary life-style, oral contraceptives (birth control pills), pregnancy (amniotic fluid emboli), long bone fractures (fat emboli), and rare blood disorders increase the risk of pulmonary emboli. (D) is incorrect because minor hand injuries usually do not cause pulmonary emboli.

333. The answer is A. (Mosby, *Medical Emergencies.*) An acute onset of pleuritic chest pain, syncope, hemoptysis, respiratory distress, hyperventilation, shock, hypotension, cardiac arrest, wheezing, and anxiety are all signs or symptoms of pulmonary embolism. Melena is a sign of gastrointestinal (GI) bleeding and is not related to pulmonary embolism.

334. The answer is C. (Mosby, *Medical Emergencies.*) (C) is the mechanism of developing a spontaneous pneumothorax. (A), (B), and (D) are all possible mechanisms of pneumothorax but not a spontaneous pneumothorax.

335. The answer is C. (Brady, *General Patient Assessment and Management.*) Acute respiratory distress, decreased or absent breath sounds on the involved side, a trachea deviated away from the involved side, distended neck veins, and hypotension are signs of a tension pneumothorax. Focal leg weakness is not related to a tension pneumothorax.

336. The answer is D. (Mosby, *Medical Emergencies.*) Paralysis, slurred speech, an altered level of consciousness, seizures, dizziness, loss of consciousness, airway problems, cardiac arrhythmias, nausea and vomiting, pupillary abnormalities, headache, and a stiff neck are all signs or symptoms of a stroke. Frequent urination is not a sign of a stroke.

337. The answer is A. (Mosby, *Medical Emergencies.*) (B), (C), and (D) demonstrate the importance of airway management in a stroke victim. (A) is incorrect because laryngitis (hoarseness) is not associated with a stroke.

338. The answer is C. (Mosby, *Medical Emergencies.*) Stroke, brain tumor, intracranial hemorrhage, CNS infections, encephalitis, meningitis, and seizures are all intracranial causes of coma. (C) is incorrect because while a narcotic overdose is a common cause of coma, it is not an intracranial cause.

339. The answer is C. (Mosby, *Medical Emergencies.*) (A), (B), (D), liver failure, a hypertensive crisis, hypothyroidism, hypoadrenalism, vitamin deficiencies, and psychiatric problems are all non–nervous system causes of coma. (C) is incorrect because ovarian failure does not cause coma.

340. Answers. (Mosby, *Medical Emergencies.*)
A = alcohol, acidosis
E = epilepsy (seizures)
I = infection
O = overdose
U = uremia (kidney failure)
T = trauma
I = insulin
P = psychosis
S = shock, stroke

341. The answer is A. (Mosby, *Medical Emergencies.*) (B), (C), (D), high-concentration O_2, frequent vital signs, preparing to suction secretions and/or vomitus, spinal immobilization, IV access with normal saline or lactated Ringer's KVO, and, if permitted by protocol, removing contact lenses are all parts of the emergency care rendered to a comatose patient. (A) is incorrect because one never administers anything orally to a comatose patient because of possible airway obstruction and/or aspiration into the lungs.

342. The answer is C. (Mosby, *Medical Emergencies.*) A generalized motor seizure, a focal motor seizure, a behavioral seizure, and status epilepticus are all types of seizure disorders. Behavioral seizures are often called petit mal in children and psychomotor seizures in adults. (C) is incorrect because there is no such diagnosis as an anxiety seizure.

343. The answer is C. (Mosby, *Medical Emergencies.*) (A), (B), (D), postictal ventilation support, postictal behavior support, pulse oximetry, and avoiding forcefully inserting bite blocks or an oral airway are all parts of the emergency care of a seizure patient. (C) is incorrect because the patient should be allowed to complete the seizure with only a soft blanket or pillow under the head. Restraining the patient is not indicated.

344. The answer is C. (Mosby, *Medical Emergencies.*) Intracranial bleeding, meningitis or encephalitis, brain tumor, a hypertensive crisis, and poisoning are some of the serious causes of headache. (C) is incorrect because anxiety frequently may cause a headache but is not a serious condition.

345. The answer is B. (Mosby, *Medical Emergencies.*) (A), (C), (D), a pneumatic antishock garment for shock, and transport in a comfortable position are all parts of the emergency care of a patient with abdominal pain. (B) is incorrect because one does not allow anything by mouth to a patient with abdominal pain.

346. The answer is B. (Mosby, *Medical Emergencies.*) Peptic ulcer disease, esophageal varices, acute gastritis, esophagitis, and stomach cancer are all causes of upper GI bleeding. (B) is incorrect because hemorrhoids are a cause of lower GI bleeding, not upper GI bleeding.

347. The answer is A. (Mosby, *Medical Emergencies.*) Colon cancer, hemorrhoids, diverticulosis, polyps, and colitis are causes of lower GI bleeding. (A) is incorrect because appendicitis is a cause of abdominal pain, not lower GI bleeding.

348. The answer is B. (Brady, *Administer 50% Dextrose.*) Palpitations, sweating, an altered level of consciousness, slurred speech, weakness, seizures, and a neurologic deficit are all signs or symptoms of hypoglycemia. Fever is not a sign or symptom of hypoglycemia.

349. The answer is D. (Mosby, *Medical Emergencies.*) (A), (B), (C), oral administration of glucose solution, candy, or corn syrup, and ECG monitoring are priorities in providing emergency care to a hypoglycemic patient. (D) is incorrect because epinephrine is not part of the emergency care of hypoglycemia.

350. The answer is A. (Mosby, *Medical Emergencies.*) (B), (C), (D), weakness, nausea and vomiting, abdominal pain, rapid deep respirations (Kussmaul's breathing), and a rapid weak pulse are all signs or symptoms of diabetic ketoacidosis. High blood pressure is incorrect because a patient in diabetic ketoacidosis usually has normal or low blood pressure.

351. The answer is A. (Mosby, *Medical Emergencies.*) Dehydration, gradual deterioration over 4 or 5 days, altered mental status, and precipitation by infection, cold, or dehydration are parts of a common presentation of hyperosmolar hyperglycemic nonketotic coma. (A) is incorrect since even though fruity breath odor is part of diabetic ketoacidosis, it is not part of the clinical presentation of hyperosmolar hyperglycemic nonketotic coma.

352. The answer is B. (Mosby, *Medical Emergencies.*) (A), (C), (D), the local protocol for drawing blood before administering IV fluids and/or medications, and checking a fingerstick glucose level are all parts of the emergency care given to a diabetic patient. (B) is incorrect because EMT-Is are not trained or authorized to administer insulin to patients.

353. The answer is A. (Mosby, *Medical Emergencies.*) Ingestion, absorption, injection, and inhalation are all routes of exposure to poison. (A) is incorrect because evaporation is a process by which the body loses water and heat. It is not related to poisoning.

354. The answer is C. (Mosby, *Medical Emergencies.*) (A), (B), (D), and a description of what has been done for the patient are important questions about a poisoned patient. (C) is incorrect, because the temperature (hot or cold) of a poison does not affect the patient's outcome.

355. The answer is D. (Mosby, *Medical Emergencies.*) Temperature, pulse, blood pressure, respiratory rate, and pupil size and reaction are important areas to check in a poisoned patient. (D) is incorrect because the presence of swollen glands has nothing to do with a poisoned patient.

356. The answer is B. (Mosby, *Medical Emergencies.*) (A), (C), and (D) are aspects of the correct use of syrup of ipecac. However, you should not induce vomiting in a patient who has an altered mental status, who has a history of seizures, who is in the third trimester of pregnancy, who has a history of cardiac disease, or who has ingested corrosives (acids or alkalis), petroleum products, iodine, strychnine, or silver nitrate. (B) is incorrect.

357. The answer is D. (Mosby, *Medical Emergencies.* Brady, *Appendix: Pulse Oximetry.*) All victims of a fire are suspected of having carbon monoxide poisoning. The EMT-I should administer high-concentration oxygen, assist ventilations if necessary, and transport the patient as soon as possible. Most inhaled poisons, including carbon monoxide, are odorless and colorless. A rapid pulse and high blood pressure are not specific signs of carbon monoxide poisoning. Usually, with carbon monoxide poisoning there is an unreliable pulse oximetry reading. The carbon monoxide attaches to hemoglobin, just as oxygen does, and causes a falsely elevated oxygen saturation value.

358. The answer is A. (Mosby, *Medical Emergencies.*) (B), (C), (D), providing high-concentration oxygen, transporting the patient to the hospital, and removing the patient to a cool environment are all parts of the emergency care. (A) is incorrect based on this description.

359. The answer is D. (Mosby, *Medical Emergencies.*) (D) is incorrect because a patient with heat exhaustion should not be allowed to take anything by mouth.

360. The answer is B. (Mosby, *Medical Emergencies.*) Rapid cooling is done by placing the patient in a cool environment; applying ice packs to the axillae, neck, wrists, and groin; and removing the patient's clothing and wrapping the patient in moist sheets. Failure to lower the patient's temperature quickly may result in permanent brain damage.

361. The answer is D. (Mosby, *Medical Emergencies.*) (A), (B), (C), covering the involved site with dry sterile dressings, checking for serious problems such as fractures and hypothermia, and not rubbing the frostbitten area with ice or snow are all parts of emergency care of frostbite. (D) is incorrect because it is very important to return a hypothermic patient's core temperature back to normal before caring for a frostbitten extremity.

362. The answer is A. (Mosby, *Medical Emergencies.*) (B), (C), (D), handling the patient gently, giving high-concentration oxygen by non-rebreather mask, and caring for other life-threatening injuries or conditions are all part of the emergency care. (A) is incorrect because in a hypothermic patient, you should check for a pulse for 30 to 45 seconds before beginning chest compressions.

OBSTETRIC
AND GYNECOLOGIC
EMERGENCIES

In this chapter, you will review:

- three stages of labor

- post-delivery complications

- care of newborn

OBSTETRIC AND GYNECOLOGIC EMERGENCIES

Directions: Each item below contains four suggested responses. Select the **one best** response to each item.

363. All of the following are the most common signs or symptoms of early pregnancy EXCEPT

(A) a missed or late menstrual period
(B) breast tenderness and enlargement
(C) nausea and vomiting
(D) burning on urination

364. All of the following are expected physiologic changes in a pregnant patient's vital signs EXCEPT

(A) temperature is always over 100° during pregnancy
(B) respiratory rate is increased
(C) resting heart rate is increased 10–20 beats per minute
(D) normal blood pressure drops 10–15 mm Hg

365. As you arrive at the side of a "sick" 8-month-pregnant 26-year-old female, a friend tells you that the patient feels dizzy whenever she lies directly on her back. As you begin to assess the patient while she is lying on her back in bed, you find her blood pressure to be 80/50 with a pulse of 110 per minute. As the patient is turned on her left side, she begins to feel better and her blood pressure increases to 110/70. This scenario best represents which of the following syndromes?

(A) The supine hypotensive syndrome
(B) A vasovagal episode
(C) Internal bleeding
(D) Abruptio placentae

366. You are dispatched to a 9-month-pregnant female who needs help delivering her baby. As you arrive on the scene, you try to determine whether the patient is in labor and whether the delivery could be imminent. All of the following are signs that this patient may be delivering her baby soon EXCEPT

(A) the patient's uterine contractions are mild in intensity, lasting about 10 seconds and occurring every 10 to 20 minutes

(B) the patient notes an urge to push either to move her bowels or to force the baby out

(C) the baby's head is "crowning," being visible at the perineum

(D) the patient's contractions may be overwhelming, and she is in "transition" and may panic and be very irritable

367. All of the following are correct statements about the three stages of labor EXCEPT

(A) the first stage proceeds from regular contractions to complete dilation of the cervix

(B) the second stage goes from complete cervical dilation to delivery of the baby

(C) the second stage usually lasts half as long as the first stage

(D) the third stage goes from "transition" to delivery of the baby

368. After one assists the mother with the delivery of a baby, all of the following are management procedures for postdelivery bleeding EXCEPT

(A) encourage the mother to breast feed

(B) massage the mother's lower abdomen

(C) apply ice packs to the perineum

(D) insert two to three sanitary napkins into the vagina

369. You have just assisted a mother in delivering a full-term baby at home. All of the following are priorities for providing newborn care EXCEPT

(A) suction the baby's nose and mouth with a bulb syringe

(B) stimulate breathing by drying the baby and rubbing the spine

(C) record the baby's APGAR scores (heart rate, respiratory rate, muscle tone, reflex irritability, and color) 5 and 10 minutes after delivery

(D) clamp the umbilical cord in two places, 6 to 9 inches from the baby, and cut between the clamps

370. After applying basic postdelivery bleeding procedures, you notice that the mother in question 369 is continuing to bleed excessively. All of the following are actions for an EMT-I to take EXCEPT

(A) administer oxygen by non-rebreather mask at 10 to 15 liters per minute
(B) continue to massage the lower abdomen to stimulate uterine contractions
(C) start an intravenous (IV) line and administer IV fluids
(D) apply ice packs to the axillae and lower back to stimulate uterine contractions

371. As you begin to assist a mother with a prehospital delivery, you notice that the baby's buttocks are presenting first, not the head. In assisting with this breech presentation delivery, all of the following should be done EXCEPT

(A) attempt to pull the baby out by the feet
(B) allow the baby's legs and trunk to deliver
(C) if the baby does not deliver within 3 minutes or begins to breathe before the head is delivered, put a gloved hand into the vagina and turn the baby's head to face the mother's back
(D) if the baby's head does not deliver within 3 minutes, transport the mother to the hospital in the knee-chest position or with her buttocks elevated

372. You are flagged down by a pedestrian to see a 9-month-pregnant female who is in labor and feels that the baby is coming. As you enter the patient's apartment, you find a 23-year-old female having a strong contraction. As you begin to assess the patient's perineum, you notice that the umbilical cord is the first presenting part in the delivery. All of the following are correct steps in managing a prolapsed cord delivery EXCEPT

(A) elevate the baby off the cord by inserting a gloved hand into the vagina and pushing on the baby's head
(B) gently push the cord back in to the vagina behind the baby's head
(C) position the mother in the knee-to-chest or head-and-torso-down position
(D) cover the exposed cord with warm, moist gauze or a cloth pad

373. You arrive at the home of a 28-year-old pregnant female who has been in labor for over 12 hours. The patient states that her contractions are lasting almost a minute and occurring every 3 to 4 minutes. Upon examination you note that the baby's arm is the first presenting part. In providing emergency care for this mother and her baby, which is the most important aspect of the care rendered by an EMT-I?

(A) Gently attempt to deliver the arm, then the shoulder, and then the other arm
(B) Carefully try to insert the arm back into the vagina
(C) Massage the lower abdomen to try to induce delivery
(D) Transport the patient to the hospital

374. You have just helped a 7-month-pregnant mother deliver a small, healthy infant, and you notice that the mother's abdomen remains unusually large. You should question and assess the patient for which of the following conditions?

(A) Multiple births
(B) Abruptio placentae
(C) Retained placenta
(D) Gas caused by constipation

375. All of the following are causes of abdominal pain in a pregnant patient EXCEPT

(A) spontaneous abortion or miscarriage
(B) abruptio placentae
(C) ectopic pregnancy
(D) pregnancy-induced hypertension

376. In addition to abruptio placentae, which of the following is a cause of vaginal bleeding in the third trimester of pregnancy?

(A) Menopause
(B) Placenta previa
(C) Breech delivery
(D) Prolapsed cord

OBSTETRIC AND GYNECOLOGIC EMERGENCIES

ANSWERS

363. **The answer is D.** (Mosby, *Ob Gyn Emergencies.*) A missed or late menstrual period, breast tenderness and enlargement, nausea and vomiting, and frequent urination are the most common signs or symptoms of early pregnancy. (D) is incorrect because burning on urination (dysuria) is a symptom of a urinary tract infection, not of early pregnancy.

364. **The answer is A.** (Mosby, *Ob Gyn Emergencies.*) (B), (C), and (D) are expected physiologic changes in a patient's vital signs during pregnancy. (A) is incorrect because a patient's temperature is not affected by pregnancy.

365. **The answer is A.** (Mosby, *Ob Gyn Emergencies.*) In the supine hypotensive syndrome, the weight of the pregnant uterus may compress the inferior vena cava, resulting in hypotension. Turning the patient on the left side will relieve this pressure on the inferior vena cava. (B) is incorrect because in a vasovagal episode the patient is hypotensive and bradycardic. (C) and (D) are incorrect because these conditions would produce hemorrhagic shock with hypotension and a rapid pulse which would not be relieved by turning the patient on the left side.

366. **The answer is A.** (Mosby, *Ob Gyn Emergencies.*) (B), (C), and (D) and ruptured membranes (bag of water) are reasonable signs that the delivery will come soon. (A) is incorrect because as labor progresses, the patient's uterine contractions become stronger, lasting 30 to 60 seconds and occurring every 2 to 3 minutes.

367. **The answer is D.** (Mosby, *Ob Gyn Emergencies.*) (A), (B), and (C) are correct. (D) is incorrect because the third stage of labor goes from the delivery of the baby to the delivery of the placenta.

368. The answer is D. (Mosby, *Ob Gyn Emergencies.*) (A), (B), (C), and applying a sanitary napkin externally to the perineum are the correct procedures. (D) is incorrect because an EMT-Intermediate (EMT-I) should never place anything within the vagina.

369. The answer is C. (Mosby, *Ob Gyn Emergencies.*) (A), (B), (D), keeping the baby warm, and recording the baby's APGAR scores after delivery are priorities for newborn care. (C) is incorrect because APGAR scores should be recorded 1 and 5 minutes after delivery.

370. The answer is D. (Mosby, *Ob Gyn Emergencies.*) (A), (B), (C), continuing to place sanitary napkins over the vagina, and applying and inflating a pneumatic antishock garment (PASG) are actions an EMT-I should take to treat excessive postdelivery bleeding. (D) is incorrect because while applying a cold pack to the perineum is part of the treatment, applying ice packs to the axillae and lower back offers no benefit.

371. The answer is A. (Mosby, *Ob Gyn Emergencies.*) (B), (C), (D), encouraging the mother to push with contractions, administering oxygen by non-rebreather mask at 10–15 liters per minute, starting an IV line, preparing to resuscitate the baby, and notifying the receiving hospital of the clinical situation are all parts of the treatment of a mother with a breech presentation.

372. The answer is B. (Mosby, *Ob Gyn Emergencies.*) (A), (C), (D), establishing IV access, administering oxygen by non-rebreather mask at 10 to 15 liters per minute, monitoring the cord for pulsations (which indicate the baby's viability), and transporting the patient rapidly are all parts of the management. (B) is incorrect because one should never push the cord back into the vagina.

373. The answer is D. (Mosby, *Ob Gyn Emergencies.*) The most important part of an EMT-I's treatment of a pregnant woman with a limb presentation is transport to the hospital. Additionally, the EMT-I should administer oxygen and start an IV line. (A), (B), and (C) are all incorrect.

374. The answer is A. (Mosby, *Ob Gyn Emergencies.*) Multiple births may be suspected when, after delivery, the mother's abdomen remains unusually large or the mother gives a history of being told of the possibility of multiple fetuses during her prenatal care. Also, multiple-birth babies are often small and deliver prematurely. Abruptio placentae usually is suspected if the patient has sudden, severe, constant lower abdominal pain; dark vaginal bleeding; and shock with a soft tender or contracting uterus. After delivery, a retained placenta and gas from constipation are not associated with an unusually large abdomen.

375. The answer is D. (Mosby, *Ob Gyn Emergencies.*) A spontaneous abortion or miscarriage, abruptio placentae, and an ectopic pregnancy are well-known causes of abdominal pain in a pregnant patient. Pregnancy-induced hypertension is not related to abdominal pain in a pregnant patient.

376. **The answer is B.** (Mosby, *Ob Gyn Emergencies.*) Placenta previa and abruptio placentae are both well-known causes of vaginal bleeding in the third trimester of pregnancy. Menopause, a breech delivery, and a prolapsed cord are not.

PEDIATRIC
EMERGENCIES

In this chapter, you will review:

- the pediatric airway

- fever in children

- common causes of pediatric trauma

PEDIATRIC EMERGENCIES

Directions: Each item below contains four suggested responses. Select the **one best** response to each item.

377. The narrowest part of a child's upper airway is the

    (A) vocal cords
    (B) oropharynx
    (C) thyroid cartilage
    (D) cricoid cartilage

378. All of the following are developmental characteristics of newborns and infants (birth to 1 year) EXCEPT that

    (A) there is minimal stranger anxiety
    (B) they are used to being undressed but like to be warm
    (C) they do not like to be separated from their parents
    (D) they readily accept an oxygen mask

379. All of the following are developmental characteristics of toddlers (ages 1 to 3 years) EXCEPT that they

    (A) are comfortable with being undressed
    (B) do not like to be touched or separated from their parents
    (C) have a fear of needles and pain
    (D) do not like being suffocated by an oxygen mask

380. All of the following are developmental characteristics of preschool children (3 to 6 years old) EXCEPT that they

    (A) are modest and do not want their clothing removed
    (B) have a fear of blood, pain, and permanent injury
    (C) are not curious, are very quiet, and rarely cooperate
    (D) do not want to be suffocated by an oxygen mask

381. All of the following are developmental characteristics of school-age children (6 to 12 years old) EXCEPT that they

(A) cooperate but like to have their opinions heard

(B) are modest and do not like to expose their bodies

(C) do not want to be suffocated by an oxygen mask

(D) fear blood, pain, disfigurement, and permanent injury

382. All of the following are developmental characteristics of adolescents (12 to 18 years old) EXCEPT that they

(A) often need to be physically restrained because of inappropriate fear of treatments

(B) want to be treated as adults

(C) often feel that they are indestructible but may fear permanent injury and disfigurement

(D) may not be comfortable exposing their changing bodies

383. All of the following are age-specific responses to illness or injury EXCEPT that

(A) newborns and infants (birth to age 1 year) are usually frightened by strangers

(B) toddlers (ages 1 to 3 years) are afraid when they are in pain or bleeding and need reassurance

(C) preschool children (ages 3 to 6 years) have active imaginations and may invent strange and frightening ideas about what is happening

(D) school-age children (ages 6 to 12 years) fear pain, blood, and permanent injury

384. All of the following are signs or symptoms of respiratory distress in infants or children EXCEPT

(A) tachypnea, nasal flaring, diminished breath sounds

(B) stridor, grunting, prolonged expirations

(C) skin rash and eye tearing

(D) decreased level of responsiveness to you, the parents, or pain

385. You arrive at a day-care center and find a 5-year-old boy who has just fallen off the monkey bars in the playground. He is crying and complaining about pain in the right leg. Your assessment reveals that the right leg is tender in the midcalf region with mild swelling, but the neurovascular function appears intact. As your partner takes the vital signs, you begin to think about the average normal vital signs for a 5-year-old child. Which of the following is correct?

(A) Pulse 120–160 per minute, respiratory rate 40–60 per minute, blood pressure 80/40

(B) Pulse 80–140 per minute, respiratory rate 30–40 per minute, blood pressure 82/44

(C) Pulse 70–115 per minute, respiratory rate 20–25 per minute, blood pressure 90/52

(D) Pulse 60–80 per minute, respiratory rate 12–20 per minute, blood pressure 120/80

386. You have been dispatched to the home of a 10-year-old girl who has been sick for over a week. The child's mother states that she has been having a fever of 103° with vomiting and diarrhea throughout the week. Her skin feels hot and dry, her tongue appears dry and caked, and her eyes appear sunken. As your partner takes this child's vital signs, you begin to recall the average normal vital signs for a 10-year-old. Which of the following is correct?

(A) Pulse 80–120 per minute, respiratory rate 25–30 per minute, blood pressure 86/50
(B) Pulse 70–115 per minute, respiratory rate 15–20 per minute, blood pressure 100/60
(C) Pulse 70–115 per minute, respiratory rate 20–25 per minute, blood pressure 94/54
(D) Pulse 70–90 per minute, respiratory rate 15–20 per minute, blood pressure 110/64

387. All of the following are the most practical methods for recalling the average normal vital signs for the pediatric age groups EXCEPT

(A) keep a reference text or table in the ambulance
(B) memorize them
(C) carry a Broselow tape with your equipment
(D) tape a table of vital signs in your drug box

388. You are dispatched to a 5-year-old boy who is having difficulty breathing. The patient's mother states that the child has had a fever with a barking cough for the past 2 days. As you immediately begin to assess the child, you note that he has stopped breathing. As you open the airway and your partner begins to perform mouth-to-mask ventilations, you reach for your airway bag to prepare for endotracheal intubation. All of the following are acceptable methods to choose the correct size endotracheal tube EXCEPT

(A) use the size of the child's external nostril as a guide
(B) select the smallest available tube and change it if necessary
(C) use the outside diameter of the child's little finger
(D) use the following formula for children over 2 years of age:

$$\text{Endotracheal tube (mm)} = \frac{\text{age in years}}{4} + 4$$

389. You are dispatched to see an unconscious child. Upon arrival, you find a 6-year-old child lying in bed with his mother crying and upset. The child's mother states that he has asthma and has been running a fever the past 3 days, with a severe cough. This morning he was noted to become weaker and very hot to touch. His mother states that she gave him only Tylenol and his inhaler. Upon assessing the child, you note that he is breathing only eight times per minute and is cyanotic. His blood pressure is 98/54, his pulse is 120 per minute, and he is very hot to touch. As you begin to assist this child's breathing, you consider the different methods of assisting with a bag-valve-mask (BVM) device. All of the following are correct statements concerning the use of the BVM in infants or children EXCEPT

    (A) in general, the BVM should provide 450 mL of volume, be attached to oxygen at 15 liters per minute, and not have a pop-off valve

    (B) in nontraumatic cases, BVM ventilation should be performed with two hands: one to hold the mask on the face and maintain the head tilt/chin lift maneuver and the other to squeeze the bag

    (C) if it is difficult to maintain a seal, it may help to invert the mask on the infant or child's face

    (D) if one EMT-Intermediate (EMT-I) is having difficulty ventilating, a two-person technique is acceptable with one EMT-I maintaining the airway while the second EMT-I maintains a tight seal on the face with the mask

390. You arrive to see a 2-year-old child with difficulty breathing. The child's mother states that the child has had a cold for the past 3 days. However, tonight the child awoke with a barking cough and some difficulty breathing. In considering the approach to a child with croup, all of the following are true EXCEPT

    (A) croup usually starts as a cold and occurs in a 3-month-old to 3-year-old child

    (B) while there may be mild respiratory distress, there is no real risk of total airway obstruction

    (C) key parts of the treatment include administering high-concentration oxygen (cool and humidified) and transporting the child in a comfortable position

    (D) the patient should be reassessed frequently for any changes in or signs of airway obstruction

391. You are dispatched to a 5-year-old boy who has fever and difficulty breathing. When you arrive, you find the child sitting on the edge of a chair in the tripod position, drooling and with stridor and in respiratory distress. This child is most likely suffering from which of the following?

    (A) Acute viral flu syndrome

    (B) Strep throat

    (C) Acute epiglottitis

    (D) Tuberculosis

392. All of the following are parts of the emergency care of a child with acute epiglottitis EXCEPT

(A) careful visualization of the throat with a tongue blade

(B) trying to keep the child calm and as comfortable as possible, preferably by having the child sit on the parent's lap

(C) high-concentration oxygen with humidification by face mask or the blow-by method

(D) being prepared to ventilate with a BVM device and perform a needle cricothyrotomy and endotracheal intubation if necessary

393. You are assigned to the home of a 6-year-old girl with acute difficulty breathing. As you enter the room, you are told that this child has a longstanding history of asthma but has begun to complain of difficulty breathing for the past hour. The child's babysitter was told that the child had a recent cold and had a little wheezing for the past 2 days. In providing emergency care for a child with an acute asthmatic attack, all of the following are true EXCEPT

(A) status asthmaticus is a life-threatening emergency, and an EMT-I must always be prepared to intubate and ventilate if necessary

(B) a severe asthmatic attack usually is manifested by loud wheezing

(C) the initial treatment includes humidified high-concentration oxygen, careful monitoring of the vital signs and cardiac rhythm, pulse oximetry, and following the local protocol

(D) the most common drug treatment provided to asthmatic patients includes bronchodilators and epinephrine

394. You are dispatched to a 1-year-old child with difficulty breathing. The child's mother, who is very upset, states that the child had a little cold for a few days but then seemed to get worse. The child initially had a little fever, a runny nose, and a cough but then seemed to be having difficulty breathing. Your assessment reveals a 1-year-old child who is tachypneic with wheezing in bilateral lung fields. In considering the possibility of bronchiolitis, you consider the treatment options available to you. All of the following are part of emergency care for bronchiolitis EXCEPT

(A) high-concentration humidified oxygen
(B) monitoring of vital signs and pulse oximetry
(C) avoiding the use of epinephrine or albuterol inhalers
(D) transport to the hospital while attempting to keep the child calm

395. All of the following are signs or symptoms of moderate to severe dehydration in an infant or child EXCEPT

(A) fever, nausea, vomiting, and diarrhea
(B) tachycardia, tachypnea, and prolonged capillary refill
(C) cool, clammy, sunken fontanelle and eyes
(D) alert with normal thirst and moist mucous membranes

396. You are performing a demonstration of EMS in your community's grammar school, when a teacher calls you for help with a 5-year-old seizing child. After a total of 10 minutes of seizing, the patient fails to become responsive before another seizure begins. This patient's clinical presentation is consistent with

(A) a focal seizure
(B) petit mal
(C) status epilepticus
(D) a simple seizure

397. All of the following are parts of the emergency treatment by an EMT-I of an infant or child with status epilepticus EXCEPT

(A) intravenous Dilantin at a dose of 15 mg/kg
(B) open and maintain the child's airway
(C) monitor cardiac activity
(D) administer intravenous (IV) glucose to correct hypoglycemia

398. You are driving to the home of a sick 1-year-old boy with fever. The child's parents say that the child developed the fever a few days ago. Since then the child has become weaker, lethargic, and irritable, with a loss of appetite and refusal of food. This morning the child developed a rash and appeared to have difficulty breathing while becoming even weaker. You suspect that this child may be suffering from

(A) a toothache
(B) an allergic reaction
(C) acute meningitis
(D) a urinary tract infection

399. In providing emergency medical care for a child with possible meningitis, all of the following are important EXCEPT

(A) monitor vital signs and cardiac status

(B) start an IV of lactated Ringer's solution and provide fluid boluses of 20 mL/kg as needed to treat shock

(C) observe closely for any signs of seizure activity

(D) use only routine body substance isolation precautions and a specialized face mask to prevent transmission of the disease

400. Which of the following statements contains the correct definition of drowning and near drowning after a submersion accident?

(A) Drowning is defined as death within 24 hours, and near drowning as survival for at least 24 hours

(B) Drowning is defined as death within 24 hours, and near drowning as survival for at least 96 hours

(C) Drowning is defined as death immediately, and near drowning as survival for at least 24 hours

(D) Drowning is defined as death within 12 hours, and near drowning as survival for at least 1 week

401. You are dispatched to a nearby lake to see a 5-year-old girl who was just pulled out of the water after being submerged for 10 to 15 minutes. As you begin to assess the child, you notice that she is very cold and has a pulse. Your emergency care should include all of the following EXCEPT

(A) remove cold, wet clothing and wrap the girl in blankets and towels

(B) perform immediate endotracheal intubation

(C) administer high-concentration oxygen

(D) supply rapid transport

402. All of the following are common poisons ingested by children in the 18-month to 3-year-old age group EXCEPT

(A) medications

(B) household products (cleaning agents, furniture polish, garden supplies)

(C) mind-altering drugs

(D) contaminated foods

403. All of the following are common poisons ingested by the school-age and adolescent age group EXCEPT

(A) household products

(B) alcohol

(C) narcotics

(D) central nervous system depressants

404. Which of the following is the correct sequence from the most common to the least common causes of pediatric trauma?

(A) Falls, accidental injury, sports-related injury, assaults, vehicular-related trauma

(B) Sports-related injury, assaults, vehicular-related trauma, falls, accidental injury

(C) Falls, vehicular-related trauma, accidental injury, sports-related injury, assaults

(D) Accidental injury, sports-related injury, falls, assaults, vehicular-related trauma

405. You are dispatched to a playground to see a 4-year-old boy who has fallen from the monkey bars and landed on his head. The child is unconscious, is breathing, and has a strong pulse. The most important intervention to be instituted in this child is

(A) immediate defibrillation with an automated external defibrillator (AED)

(B) nasotracheal intubation

(C) IV line and fluid administration

(D) establishment of an airway and provision of ventilation with BVM or endotracheal intubation

406. You are dispatched to a child who has been struck by a motor vehicle. As you arrive at the scene, a witness states that this 3-year-old child was on his bike when he was hit broadside by a car. The child was thrown 15 feet in the air and then landed on the street. All of the following are parts of the process of pediatric spinal immobilization EXCEPT

(A) initially, manually hold the child's head in a neutral in-line position

(B) apply a rigid cervical collar only if it fits properly

(C) logroll the child onto a rigid board and fasten the torso and then the head to the spinal board

(D) gently lie the spinal board on the top of the stretcher and immediately begin transport

407. All of the following are possible signs of blunt abdominal trauma in a pediatric patient EXCEPT

(A) abdominal distention, rigidity, or tenderness

(B) signs of unexplained shock

(C) upper chest skin bruising from a shoulder-chest safety belt

(D) an unstable pelvis

408. You are dispatched to a ski lodge where a father and his 10-year-old son have been brought after a serious skiing accident. The father has multiple fractures and a head injury and is being taken care of by a paramedic unit from town. You are asked to take care of the 10-year-old boy, who was not injured but remained out in the cold snow with his father for over 3.5 hours. On examination, the child is becoming more lethargic, is breathing six times a minute, and has a pulse of 40 per minute. All of the following are parts of providing emergency care to this hypothermic child EXCEPT

(A) move the patient to a warmer environment right away

(B) remove all wet clothing, wrap the patient in blankets, and cover the patient's head

(C) maintain the airway and provide 100% oxygen by face mask

(D) put heat packs directly on the skin in bilateral axillae

409. You are dispatched to a house where a child has been injured, and a neighbor has called in to note that child abuse may be involved in this case. As you drive to the scene, you think of the various signs of child abuse. All of the following are possible signs EXCEPT

(A) injuries in various stages of healing or scattered on many parts of the body

(B) a smiling child, well nourished, who was injured while playing outside with his or her friends

(C) a child who appears malnourished, dirty, very withdrawn and quiet

(D) any obvious or suspected fracture in a child under 2 years of age

410. Which of the following is the most consistent finding in a child with a cognitive disability?

(A) The physical examination is usually dramatically abnormal

(B) Usually there is focal weakness in an extremity

(C) There is a difference between the child's level of understanding and his or her ability to communicate

(D) There are visual and auditory deficiencies

411. All of the following are suggestive of a child's having a physical disability EXCEPT

(A) the child has a large skin rash

(B) the child uses a wheelchair, crutches, or braces

(C) the child's parent describes a history of a birth defect, spinal cord injury or severe injury, or infection

(D) the child demonstrates a dramatic inability to perform a normal physical motion without any sign of an acute injury

412. You are dispatched to a pediatric skilled nursing facility to see a 3-year-old child with difficulty breathing caused by an occluded tracheostomy tube. As you arrive at the child's bedside, you find a smaller than expected child breathing 42 times per minute with supraclavicular and intercostal retractions. As you inspect the child's neck, you find a small tracheostomy tube with very little air exchange. All of the following are parts of providing emergency care for a child with an occluded tracheostomy tube EXCEPT

(A) initially, the EMT-I should remove the tracheostomy tube

(B) after removing the occluded tracheostomy tube, the EMT-I should suction the stoma and attempt to insert a new tracheostomy tube (if available) or an infant endotracheal tube

(C) if the EMT-I is unable to ventilate the patient through the stoma and the upper airway is patent, after the stoma has been occluded, a bag-valve-mask should be placed over the nose and face

(D) if bag-valve-mask ventilation is successful, orotracheal intubation should be performed or a new tracheostomy tube (if available) should be inserted

413. You have been dispatched to the home of a 5-year-old child with a disability who is sick with fever, nausea, and vomiting. As you arrive in the child's home, you find the parents providing care and comfort for the child. In evaluating a child with a disability, you recall certain considerations for the family in providing emergent care. All of the following are appropriate parts of this care EXCEPT

(A) the first step is to be assertive in requesting that the family members be removed to another room so that you and your partner can care for the child

(B) the scene may be fairly emotional for the child's entire family because of fairly frequent urgencies and/or emergencies for the child

(C) if possible, the siblings of the child should be included in providing the treatment of this patient

(D) if they prefer to do so, the family members should be included in providing the treatment of this patient

PEDIATRIC EMERGENCIES

A N S W E R S

377. The answer is D. (Brady, *Airway Management and Ventilation.*) An uncuffed endotracheal tube is used to intubate infants and children less than 8 years of age because of the narrowing of the upper airway at the cricoid cartilage.

378. The answer is D. (AAOS, *Infant and Child Emergency Care.* Westfal, *PreTest EMT-Basic.*) (A), (B), and (C) are all correct. Also, younger infants follow movement with their eyes; older infants are more active, having developed a personality. (D) is incorrect because infants do not want to be suffocated by an oxygen mask.

379. The answer is A. (AAOS, *Infant and Child Emergency Care.* Westfal, *PreTest EMT-Basic.*) (B), (C), and (D) are all correct. Toddlers also frighten easily, begin to assert their independence, and may believe that an illness is a punishment for being bad. (A) is incorrect because toddlers do not like having their clothes removed.

380. The answer is C. (AAOS, *Infant and Child Emergency Care.* Westfal, *PreTest EMT-Basic.*) (A), (B), and (D) are all correct. Preschoolers also do not like to be touched or separated from their parents. They also may believe that an illness is a punishment for being bad. (C) is incorrect; preschoolers are usually curious and communicative and may be cooperative.

381. The answer is C. (AAOS, *Infant and Child Emergency Care.* Westfal, *PreTest EMT-Basic.*) School-age children will often accept an oxygen mask if one takes the time to explain its use.

382. The answer is A. (AAOS, *Infant and Child Emergency Care.* Westfal, *PreTest EMT-Basic.*) Adolescents do not require physical restraints for emergency care treatment.

However, while they prefer to be treated as adults, they often need as much support and reassurance as children do.

383. The answer is A. (AAOS, *Infant and Child Emergency Care.* Westfal, *PreTest EMT-Basic.*) Newborns and infants usually are not frightened by strangers. The other choices are true. Adolescents (ages 12 to 18) are very concerned about permanent injury and how they will look as a result.

384. The answer is C. (Mosby, *Pediatric Emergencies.*) (A); (B); (D); poor skeletal tone; cyanosis; head bobbing; intercostal, subcostal, and suprasternal retractions; and a slow or irregular respiratory rate are all signs or symptoms of respiratory distress in infants or children. A skin rash and eye tearing are not.

385. The answer is C. (Mosby, *Pediatric Emergencies.*) (A) gives the average normal vital signs for a newborn. (B) gives the average normal vital signs for a 1-year-old child. (D) gives the average normal vital signs for an adult.

386. The answer is B. (Mosby, *Pediatric Emergencies.*) (A) gives the average normal vital signs for a 3-year-old child. (C) gives the average normal vital signs for a 7-year-old child. (D) gives the average normal vital signs for a 15-year-old adolescent.

387. The answer is B. (Mosby, *Pediatric Emergencies.*) (A), (C), and (D) are all practical methods of recalling the vital signs for the various pediatric age groups. (B) is an option but is not very practical.

388. The answer is B. (Mosby, *Pediatric Emergencies.*) (A), (C), and (D) are all acceptable methods of selecting the endotracheal tube size for this child. (B) is incorrect.

389. The answer is D. (Mosby, *Pediatric Emergencies.*) (D) is incorrect because in using the two-person technique, one EMT-I maintains the airway and mask seal on the face while the second EMT-I ventilates the patient.

390. The answer is B. (Mosby, *Pediatric Emergencies.*) (B) is incorrect because every child with croup is at risk of complete airway obstruction from worsening subglottic and vocal cord edema.

391. The answer is C. (Mosby, *Pediatric Emergencies.*) While acute viral flu syndrome and strep throat can cause fever, sore throat, and hoarseness, they should not cause drooling, tripod positioning, or respiratory distress. Tuberculosis is uncommon in children and does not present with the clinical picture described here.

392. The answer is A. (Mosby, *Pediatric Emergencies.*) (B), (C), (D), and providing notification to the receiving hospital are all parts of the emergency care. (A) is incorrect because in a child with possible epiglottitis one should never put anything in the patient's mouth or try to visualize the airway.

393. The answer is B. (Mosby, *Pediatric Emergencies.*) (A), (C), and (D) are part of the emergency care. (B) is incorrect because the most severe asthmatic attacks often present with no wheezing, with a silent chest. This child may be moving very little air and may soon progress to respiratory failure and/or respiratory arrest.

394. The answer is C. (Mosby, *Pediatric Emergencies.*) (A), (B), and (D) are all parts of the emergency care for bronchiolitis. (C) is incorrect because epinephrine and albuterol are used as treatment options for a child with bronchiolitis. However, because bronchiolitis is caused by a virus, these medications are not always effective.

395. The answer is D. (Mosby, *Pediatric Emergencies.*) (D) is incorrect because these are normal signs or symptoms. However, with mild dehydration, an infant or child may be alert.

396. The answer is C. (Mosby, *Pediatric Emergencies.*) (C) is correct. A focal seizure presents with tonic or clonic contractions in one part of the body. Petit mal is manifested by a short period of losing consciousness, often with staring off into space. A simple seizure is usually isolated, or if it recurs, there is a lucid interval before the next one.

397. The answer is A. (Mosby, *Pediatric Emergencies.*) (B), (C), and (D) are parts of the emergency treatment of pediatric status epilepticus. (A) is incorrect because even though intravenous Dilantin is part of the emergency treatment of status epilepticus, it is not administered by an EMT-I.

398. The answer is C. (Mosby, *Pediatric Emergencies.*) Meningitis should be suspected from this clinical presentation. An older child may present with headache, stiff neck, and/or Kernig's sign (pain with leg extension). Parts of the clinical presentation may fit (A), (B), and (D), but the entire picture does not.

399. The answer is D. (Mosby, *Pediatric Emergencies.*) (A), (B), and (C) are correct. (D) is incorrect because in using body isolation precautions, any face mask can provide a barrier between the EMT-I and the patient's respiratory secretions.

400. The answer is A. (Mosby, *Pediatric Emergencies.*) (A) is the correct answer even if the child eventually dies.

401. The answer is B. (Mosby, *Pediatric Emergencies.*) (A), (C), and (D) are correct. (B) is incorrect because this patient should have assisted ventilation with a BVM. Invasive procedures such as endotracheal intubation cause stimulation of the vagus nerve and may cause asystole.

402. The answer is C. (Mosby, *Pediatric Emergencies.*) Medications, household products, contaminated foods, and toxic plants are common poisons ingested by children in this age group. Mind-altering drugs are commonly ingested by the school-age through adolescent age group.

403. The answer is A. (Mosby, *Pediatric Emergencies.*) Alcohol, narcotics, central nervous system depressants, organic solvents, and mind-altering drugs are commonly ingested by this age group. Household products are commonly ingested in the 18-month to 3-year age group.

404. The answer is C. (Mosby, *Pediatric Emergencies.*) (C) is the correct sequence.

405. The answer is D. (Mosby, *Pediatric Emergencies.*) (D) is the correct answer. (A) is incorrect because the child has a pulse and should not be attached to an AED or defibrillated. (B) is incorrect because a patient with head trauma should not be intubated by the nasotracheal method. If there is a cribriform plate fracture at the base of the skull, an attempt at nasotracheal intubation may result in placement of the endotracheal tube into the brain. (C) is incorrect because airway and ventilation are of primary importance. IV and fluid administration is a lesser priority.

406. The answer is D. (Mosby, *Pediatric Emergencies.*) (D) is incorrect because after the child has been secured to the spinal board, the board must be secured to the stretcher before transport is provided.

407. The answer is C. (Mosby, *Pediatric Emergencies.*) (A), (B), and (D) are correct. (C) is incorrect because abdominal skin bruising from a lap safety belt is a sign of blunt abdominal trauma, not chest skin bruising.

408. The answer is D. (Mosby, *Pediatric Emergencies.*) (A), (B), and (C) are correct. If the child is responsive, you also may give him or her warm liquids to drink. (D) is incorrect because heat packs may be applied to bilateral axillae and the groin, but only if they do not directly touch the skin. You should wrap them first in a towel or blanket.

409. The answer is B. (Mosby, *Pediatric Emergencies.*) (A), (C), (D), more injuries than usually are seen in other children of a similar age, bruises or burns in a pattern suggesting intentional infliction, suspected increased intracranial pressure in an infant, suspected intraabdominal trauma in a young child, an injury not fitting the description of the cause, any child accused of self-injury, long-standing skin infections, inappropriate clothing for the situation, and a child who withdraws from a parent are possible signs of child abuse. (B) is not a sign of child abuse.

410. The answer is C. (Mosby, *Pediatric Emergencies.*) (A), (B), and (D) are incorrect because each is an example of a physical disability.

411. **The answer is A.** (Mosby, *Pediatric Emergencies.*) (B), (C), and (D) are correct. (A) is incorrect because a skin rash is not a sign of a physical disability.

412. **The answer is A.** (Mosby, *Pediatric Emergencies.*) (B), (C), and (D) are correct. (A) is incorrect because initially, the EMT-I should attempt to suction an occluded tracheostomy tube. Mucous plugging is the most common cause of occlusion.

413. **The answer is A.** (Mosby, *Pediatric Emergencies.*) (B), (C), and (D) are correct. (A) is incorrect because the family members are usually so involved in the care of the child that they have become experts in dealing with the child and his or her disability. The child and the family will benefit from being included in the emergent treatment as well.

SUBSTANCE ABUSE AND BEHAVIORAL EMERGENCIES

In this chapter, you will review:

- presenting alcoholic conditions

- neurotic vs. psychotic episodes

- signs of depression

SUBSTANCE ABUSE AND BEHAVIORAL EMERGENCIES

Directions: Each item below contains four suggested responses. Select the **one best** response to each item.

414. All of the following are medical conditions which may mimic alcohol intoxication EXCEPT

(A) drug abuse
(B) hypoglycemia
(C) head injury
(D) renal colic

415. You are dispatched to a 50-year-old alcoholic with the shakes. As you arrive at the patient's apartment, his wife states that he has been a very heavy drinker (more than a dozen beers and a pint of whiskey daily for the past 8 years) who decided to stop drinking 3 days ago. After examining the patient, you note that he is tremulous, tachycardic, and hypertensive. In trying to anticipate a serious clinical sign of alcohol withdrawal syndrome, you prepare to TREAT

(A) swollen ankles
(B) seizures
(C) a skin infection (cellulitis)
(D) diarrhea

416. All of the following are major classes of abused drugs EXCEPT

(A) narcotics
(B) stimulants
(C) hallucinogens
(D) anti-inflammatories

417. You are returning from the gas station and are waved down by a frantic teenage boy. He is yelling that his brother has taken some drugs and cannot be woken up. As you run upstairs to his room, you find a 17-year-old male who is unresponsive with saliva coming out of his mouth. All of the following are part of the emergency care provided to patients suspected of alcohol or drug abuse EXCEPT

(A) maintain the airway, give nasal oxygen 3 to 4 liters per minute, use an electrocardiogram monitor, and start an intravenous (IV) line
(B) prepare to suction if vomiting begins
(C) contact medical control or follow medical protocols for administering IV 50% dextrose and/or IV naloxone
(D) immediately administer syrup of ipecac

418. Which of the following is the correct definition of a behavioral emergency?

(A) An individual performs an act which is socially or morally inappropriate
(B) There is a situation in which an individual's behavior is judged to be illegal
(C) A patient feels that he or she has lost control of his or her life
(D) An individual's behavior is judged to be emergently upsetting to his or her family

419. You are called to treat an emotionally disturbed person. As you enter the apartment, you notice two individuals talking with a very upset and agitated 40-year-old male. All of the following are parts of the general approach to treating a patient with a behavioral emergency EXCEPT

(A) proceed with assertive measures by insisting that the patient calm down now
(B) allow the patient to express any feelings of anger and frustration
(C) maintain an open exit for the EMT-I and the patient
(D) avoid extended eye contact

420. As you begin to interact with an emotionally disturbed patient, you are trying to decide whether the patient is suffering from a neurotic or a psychotic episode. What is the main difference between these two conditions?

(A) A neurosis is an abnormal anxiety reaction to a perceived fear, while a psychosis is a severe anxiety reaction

(B) A neurosis is an abnormal anxiety reaction to a nonexistent situation, while a psychosis is a series of inappropriate statements

(C) A neurosis is an abnormal anxiety reaction to a perceived fear, while a psychosis exists when a patient has no concept of reality and believes that his or her imagined situation is real

(D) A neurosis is an abnormal anxiety reaction to a perceived fear, while a psychosis exists when a patient expresses overwhelming anger and frustration at an upsetting episode

421. All of the following are signs of depression EXCEPT

(A) stuttering speech

(B) an unkempt appearance

(C) frequent crying episodes

(D) an abnormally increased or decreased appetite

SUBSTANCE ABUSE AND BEHAVIORAL EMERGENCIES

ANSWERS

414. **The answer is D.** (Mosby, *Substance Abuse and Behavioral Emergencies.*) Drug abuse, hypoglycemia, head injury, brain tumor, meningitis, stroke, a postictal state, diabetic ketoacidosis, and hypoxia are all medical conditions which may mimic alcohol intoxication. (D) is not.

415. **The answer is B.** (Mosby, *Substance Abuse and Behavioral Emergencies.*) Alcohol withdrawal seizures constitute a serious clinical finding. Delirium tremens is a potentially life-threatening alcohol withdrawal syndrome, consisting of delirium, hallucinations, fear, tachycardia, and hypertension. Swollen ankles, a skin infection, and diarrhea are found commonly in alcoholics but are not related to alcohol withdrawal and usually are not serious.

416. **The answer is D.** (Mosby, *Substance Abuse and Behavioral Emergencies.*) Narcotics, stimulants, hallucinogens, depressants, and volatile chemicals are major classes of abused drugs. Anti-inflammatories are not commonly abused drugs.

417. **The answer is D.** (Mosby, *Substance Abuse and Behavioral Emergencies.*) (A), (B), (C), monitoring for shock, and restraining the patient from hurting himself or herself are parts of the emergency care of alcohol or drug abuse. (D) is incorrect because most emergency medical service (EMS) physicians do not prescribe ipecac in the prehospital or hospital setting. Also, even if ipecac was being considered by the EMT-Intermediate (EMT-I) and the medical control physician, it is never ordered in an unresponsive patient because of the high probability of aspiration and inability to protect the airway.

418. **The answer is C.** (Mosby, *Substance Abuse and Behavioral Emergencies.*) (C) is the correct definition. (A), (B), and (D) are not correct.

419. The answer is A. (Mosby, *Substance Abuse and Behavioral Emergencies.*) (B), (C), (D), having physical assistance nearby in the prehospital setting, and forming an alliance with the patient and trying to understand how the patient feels are all parts of the general approach. (A) is incorrect because the EMT-I must try to calm and soothe a patient with a behavioral emergency.

420. The answer is C. (Mosby, *Substance Abuse and Behavioral Emergencies.*) (C) is the correct answer. A psychotic patient may hear voices as well.

421. The answer is A. (Mosby, *Substance Abuse and Behavioral Emergencies.*) An unkempt appearance, frequent crying episodes, an abnormally increased or decreased appetite, speaking in short monotonic phrases without any spark or enthusiasm, and sleep disturbances are all signs of depression. A depressed patient may be able to get to sleep but often awakens in a few hours and is unable to return to sleep.

BIBLIOGRAPHY

Bledsoe BE, Cherry RA, Porter RS: *Intermediate Emergency Care*. Upper Saddle River, NJ, Brady, 1995.

Crosby LA, Lewallen DG (eds.): *Emergency Care and Transportation of the Sick and Injured,* 6/e. Chicago, American Academy of Orthopedic Surgeons (AAOS), 1995.

Shade B, Rothenberg MA, Wertz E, Jones S: *Mosby's EMT-Intermediate Textbook*. St. Louis, Mosby-Lifeline, 1997.

Westfal RE, Filangeri J: *PreTest: EMT-Basic: Self-Assessment and Review*. New York, McGraw-Hill, 1998.

ISBN 0-07-069636-5

90000

9 780070 696365